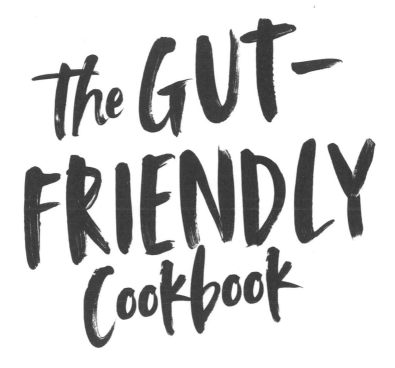

The GUT-FRIENDLY Cookbook

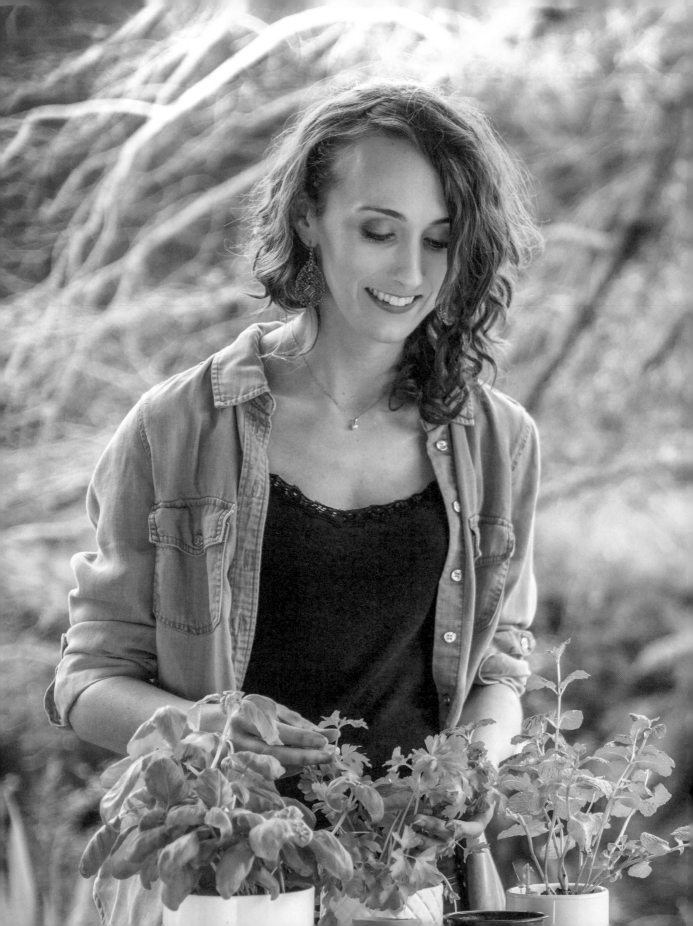

Delicious, Low-FODMAP, Gluten-Free,
Allergy-Friendly Recipes for a Happy Tummy

The GUT-FRIENDLY Cookbook

ALANA SCOTT

THE COUNTRYMAN PRESS
A division of W. W. Norton & Company
Independent Publishers Since 1923

Text copyright © 2019 by Alana Scott
Photography copyright © 2019 by Alana Scott, except pages 2, 6–7, 8 (top right and bottom left), 11, 12–13, 14, 32–33, 60–61, 100–101, 127, 152–153, 186–187, 189, 195, 197, 218, 220 copyright © by Vanessa Lewis
Design by Cat Taylor © Penguin Random House New Zealand

First American edition 2019

For information about permission to reproduce selections from this book, write to Permissions, The Countryman Press, 500 Fifth Avenue, New York, NY 10110

For information about special discounts for bulk purchases, please contact W. W. Norton Special Sales at specialsales@wwnorton.com or 800-233-4830

Manufacturing by ToppanLeefung

The Countryman Press
www.countrymanpress.com

A division of W. W. Norton & Company, Inc.
500 Fifth Avenue, New York, NY 10110
www.wwnorton.com

Library of Congress Cataloging-in-Publication Data

Names: Scott, Alana, author.
Title: The gut-friendly cookbook : delicious low-fodmap, gluten-free, allergy-friendly recipes for a happy tummy / Alana Scott.
Description: First American edition. | New York, NY : The Countryman Press, 2019. | Includes bibliographical references and index.
Identifiers: LCCN 2019045423 | ISBN 9781682684917 (paperback) | ISBN 9781682684924 (ebook)
Subjects: LCSH: Irritable colon—Diet therapy—Recipes. | Malabsorption syndromes—Diet therapy—Recipes. | LCGFT: Cookbooks.
Classification: LCC RC862.I77 S295 2019 | DDC 641.5/63—dc23
LC record available at https://lccn.loc.gov/2019045423

10 9 8 7 6 5 4 3

Thank You

I need to give a huge thank you to Toby, Tim, and my mom, Linda. Without you this book would never have been possible. I also want to thank my friends, fans, dietitian team, and mentors for inspiring me, challenging me, and always believing in me.

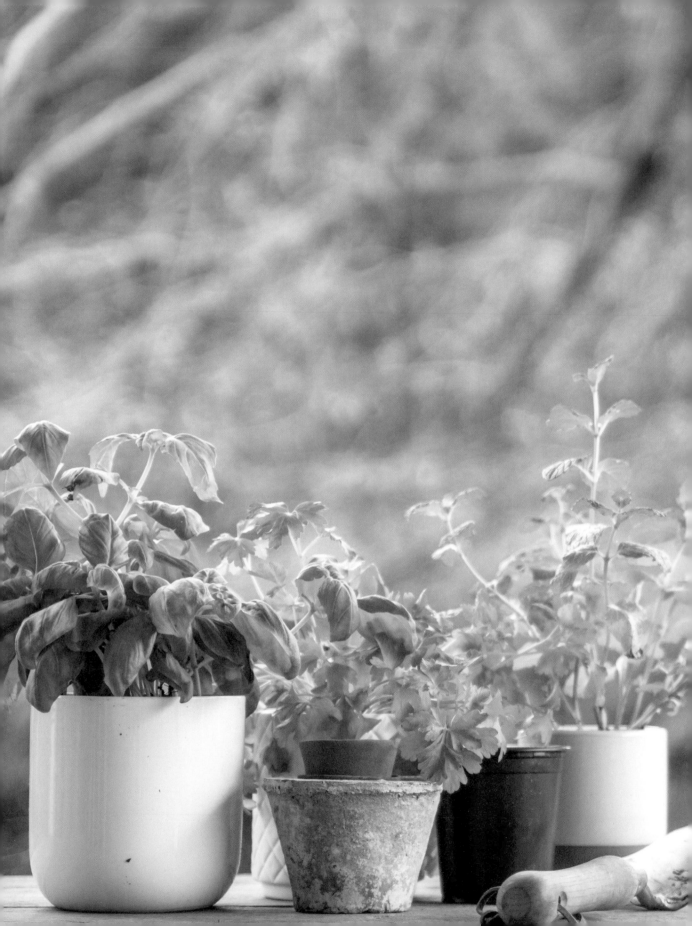

Contents

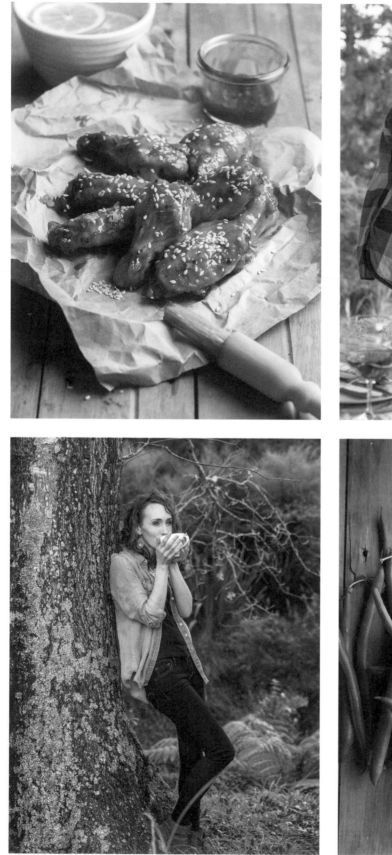
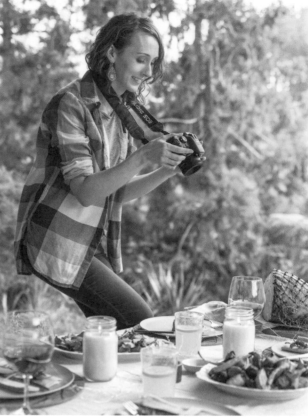
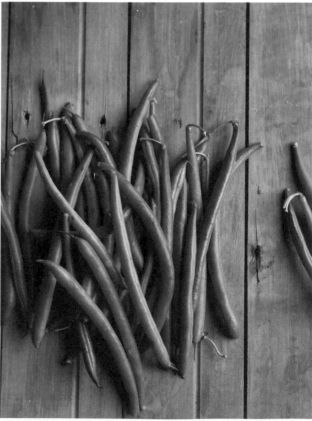

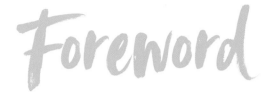
Foreword

As a gut health expert dietitian, I know how debilitating and miserable it can be living with irritable bowel syndrome (IBS) symptoms. For the 15 percent of us who suffer from embarrassing, painful, and unpredictable gut upset, a simple food choice can ruin our day. But, as a FODMAP expert dietitian, I also know that it doesn't have to be this way!

The good news is that for 75 percent of us, the low-FODMAP diet has been scientifically proven to make pain, bloating, and misery resolve in a matter of days. To date, it is the most well-researched and effective method of managing IBS-type symptoms. In fact, when implemented with the guidance and support of a specialized registered dietitian, this diet can almost be like a magic wand.

Part of the challenge I have with my patients is helping them fall back in love with food while avoiding misinformation about the low-FODMAP diet. After working with Alana over the past few years, I know that when I recommend her recipes, my patients are not only getting great food, but are also getting credible, accurate, and up-to-date information.

I love that Alana and I agree that good food doesn't need to be complicated or difficult, and that the best meals are always the ones that are simple to prepare and good to eat. *The Gut-Friendly Cookbook* fits this brief perfectly. It's full of easy, fuss-free, low-FODMAP meals that are yummy to eat and that will leave your gut feeling great, too.

If you're ready to be in charge of your gut, then take back control and add this cookbook to your IBS toolbox. It's the perfect guide to help you settle your symptoms throughout phase one of the low-FODMAP diet and get you ready to pinpoint your individual triggers through structured challenges in phase two.

We don't want you to just survive—we want you to thrive!

Joanna Baker
Accredited Practicing Dietitian
Everyday Nutrition—The Gut Health Experts

everyday nutrition

Alana has been a generous long-term supporter of Allergy New Zealand, and we were very happy to review the recipes for her cookbook. For many of those affected by food allergies or intolerances, this cookbook will be a delight.

Penny Jorgensen
Allergy New Zealand Inc., New Zealand's national allergy charity

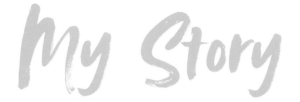

My Story

HEY FRIENDS!

I'm so excited to be releasing my first cookbook! Over the past few years I have loved hearing your stories and supporting you on your health journeys, through alittlebityummy.com. This book contains everything I wish I had known before starting my low-FODMAP journey, as well as my favorite recipes. I hope it helps you embrace your food intolerances and learn to love your food again.

My journey began when I was at university studying for my business management degree. I was into everything and loving life. My friends saw me as a kind, caring, Type A personality who had her life together.

What they didn't know was that I was the girl sitting in the middle of a crowded lecture sneakily unzipping her tight skinny jeans to let her bloated belly escape. I was also the girl who would stand in the corner of networking events trying to have a sneaky fart while praying that no one would decide it's time to chat. And the girl who would race to the bathroom and bang on occupied toilet doors while doing the "I need to poop" two-step. Eventually, I became the girl who felt too ill to leave the house.

When I confessed to my doctor what was going on, I was referred to a gastroenterologist and dietitian from whom I received a diagnosis of celiac disease and then irritable bowel syndrome (IBS). A strict gluten-free diet for my celiac disease was not enough to settle my symptoms, so I was also placed on a low-FODMAP diet.

My initial thought was FOD-what? The low-FODMAP diet sounded complex and overwhelming. My dietitian was sure the diet could help but I wasn't sure how I was going to survive on it.

My first trip to the supermarket was tragic. I remember trudging around the store crying while my mom flicked through multiple pieces of paper trying to figure out what I could eat. I left the store that afternoon with a bag of carrots and a chicken breast, feeling like I was doomed to a lifetime of boring meals.

Once home I had a choice to make: to sit there and feel sorry for myself or to make the low-FODMAP diet work for me. I decided that I never wanted anyone to feel so lonely or defeated starting their FODMAP journey, so I founded *A Little Bit Yummy*.

My foodie background, from growing up in a country restaurant nestled on our deer farm, my basic cooking skills, and my problem-solving ability all came in handy as I got stuck into cooking lo-fo style. We had a few disasters, like the time I set the oven on fire while cooking a lamb roast . . . but for the most part, the meals were a success and my friends and family didn't even notice they were eating low FODMAP.

The even better news is that my IBS symptoms decreased by more than 80 percent and I felt human again. To this day, I am on a modified FODMAP diet where I eat a lot of low-FODMAP foods and enjoy small amounts of high-FODMAP foods that don't trigger my symptoms.

A Little Bit Yummy now helps hundreds of thousands of people around the world by providing dietitian-approved low-FODMAP resources. I can't wait to guide you through the low-FODMAP diet and to help you gain good symptom management.

Happy eating!

—Alana

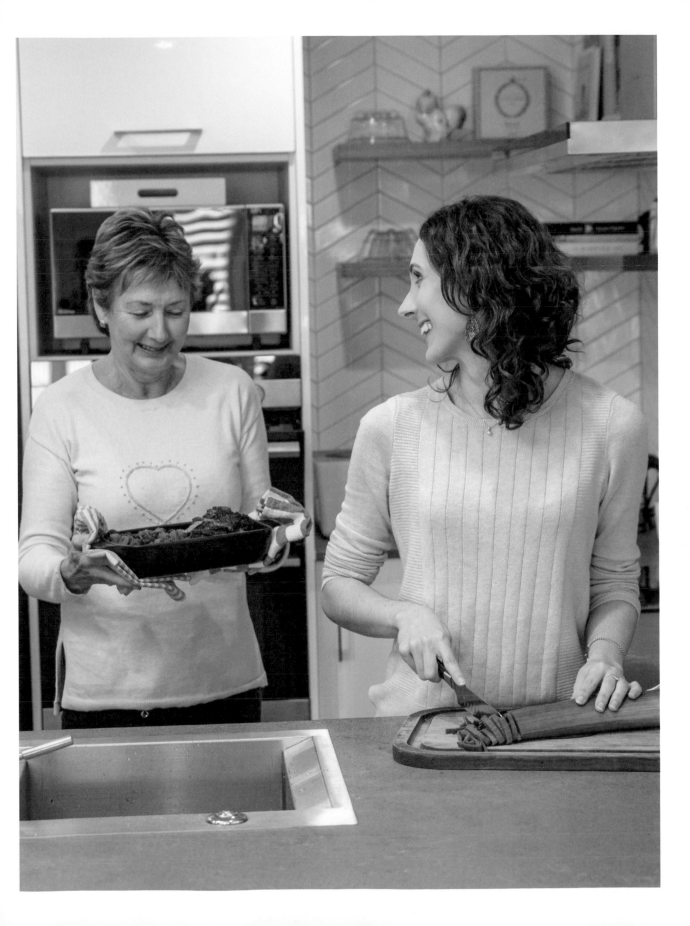

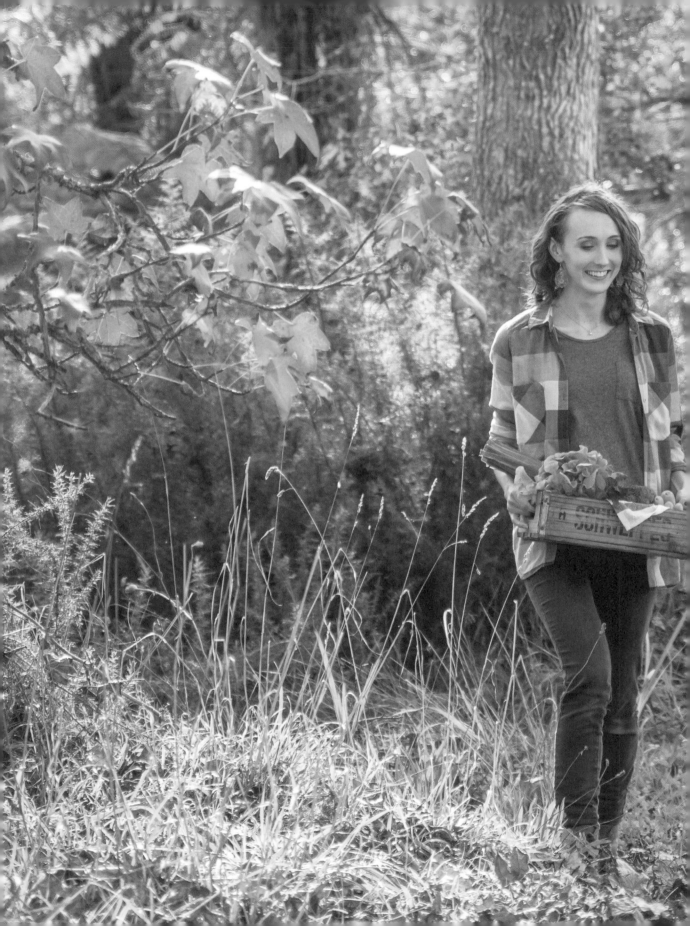

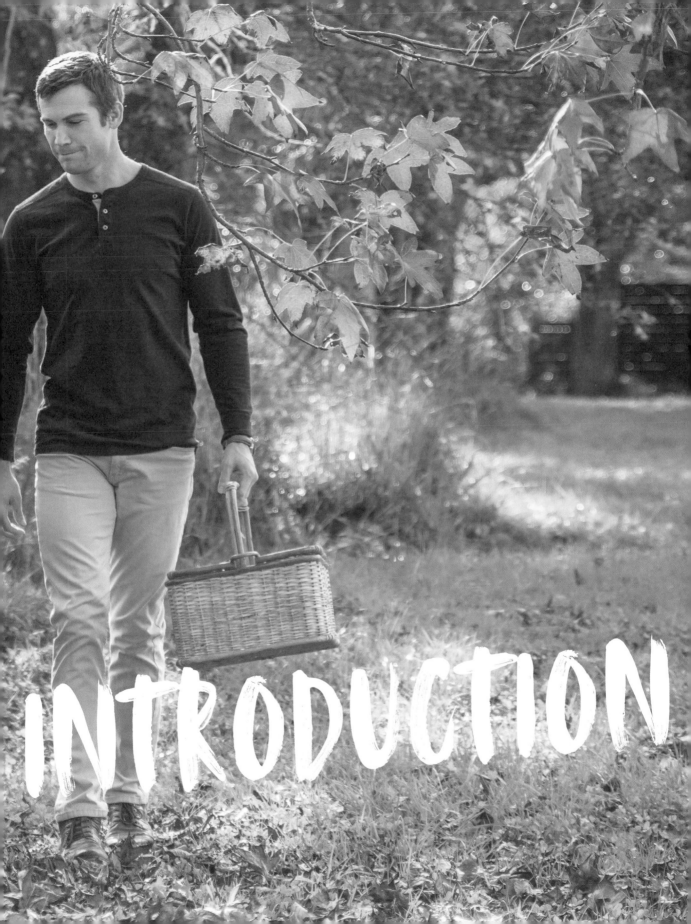

INTRODUCTION

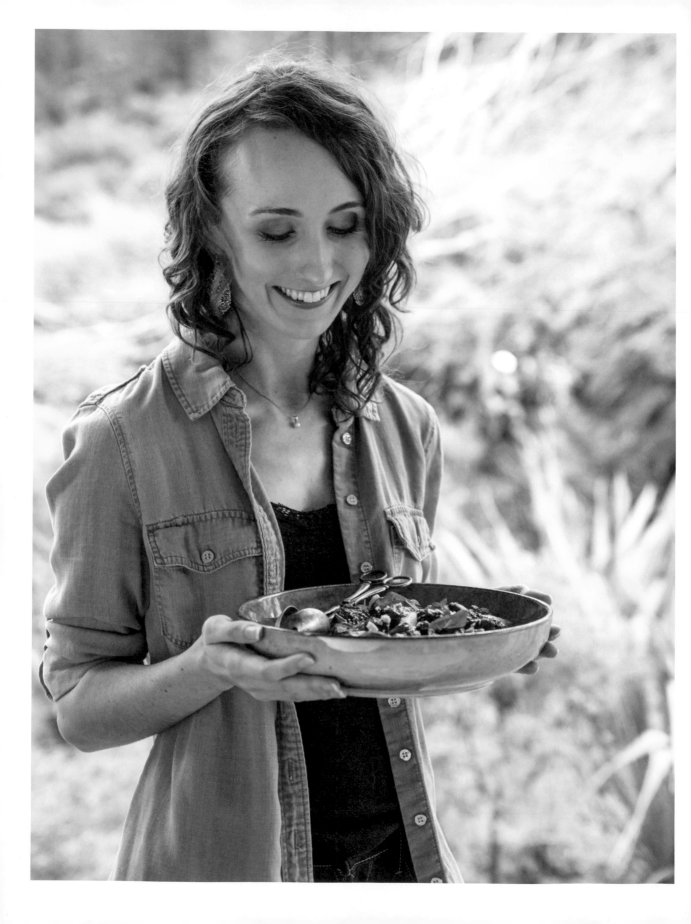

FODMAP Basics

IS THE LOW-FODMAP DIET RIGHT FOR YOU?

The low-FODMAP diet has been designed as a tool that can help up to 75 percent of irritable bowel syndrome (IBS) sufferers gain good symptom management, through identifying foods that trigger symptoms. This statistic is exciting, and I know it's tempting to plunge straight into the low-FODMAP diet, but it's important that you check first whether it's right for you.

BEFORE YOU START

- Check with your doctor before changing your diet and get a clear diagnosis. Make sure your doctor has ruled out celiac disease (you need to be eating gluten for these tests), inflammatory bowel disease, and bowel cancer, as these conditions can have similar symptoms to IBS.
- If you have other medical conditions, ask if the low-FODMAP diet is a suitable symptom-management option.
- Get a referral to a FODMAP-trained dietitian. The low-FODMAP diet is a restrictive medical diet and it's important that you have a dietitian who can help guide you and tailor the diet to your needs.
- If you have an eating disorder, use food for emotional support, or are obsessive about your food, then the low-FODMAP diet might not be right for you and you need to seek specialized medical advice.
- Check with a medical professional before placing children, elderly people, or pregnant women on the diet as these groups all have different nutritional needs to support their bodies. The low-FODMAP diet is a restrictive diet and may not be appropriate.
- Make sure you are able and prepared to restrict your diet for a two- to six-week period while you see if the diet helps you gain good symptom management.
- Be mentally prepared to reintroduce some high-FODMAP foods back into your diet after two to six weeks to support your long-term gut health.

WHAT ARE FODMAPS?

In really simple terms, FODMAP is an acronym that represents a group of fermentable sugars (short-chain carbohydrates) that are found in a wide range of foods and can trigger unpleasant gastrointestinal symptoms in some people. Let's break down the acronym:

Fermentable: The process through which gut bacteria break down undigested carbohydrates and produce gases (hydrogen, methane, and carbon dioxide) as a side effect.

Oligosaccharides: There are two main types of oligosaccharides. The first type is fructo-oligosaccharides (FOS or fructans), found in foods such as wheat, rye, onions, and garlic. The second type is galacto-oligosaccharides (GOS or galactans), found in legumes and pulses. Have you ever wondered where the saying "beans means farts" came from? A fun fact is that humans aren't actually designed to be able to break down oligosaccharides and this is why they can make everyone windy. Unfortunately, for those of us with a sensitive gut, this is more painful than it is for others.

Disaccharides: The only disaccharide classified as a FODMAP is lactose. Lactose contains two sugar units that need to be separated by an enzyme called lactase. If you don't have enough lactase enzymes, your body won't be able to separate the sugar units and you will malabsorb lactose. Lactose is found in milk, soft cheese (e.g. ricotta), yogurt, and ice cream.

Monosaccharides: Fructose is a monosaccharide. Because glucose can help your body absorb fructose by acting as a "co-transporter," only excess fructose is considered high-FODMAP. When you consume more fructose than glucose, your body may not be able to effectively process the fructose, resulting in malabsorption, which can trigger symptoms. High-FODMAP foods that contain excess fructose include honey, mango, apples, pears, and high-fructose corn syrup.

And Polyols: Polyols are sugar alcohols that are found naturally in some fruit and vegetables. They can also be man-made and used as artificial sweeteners. These sugar alcohols won't make you drunk but they are incompletely absorbed across the small intestine, which is why they can cause gastrointestinal symptoms. Polyols include mannitol and sorbitol. Grab the Monash University Low-FODMAP Diet™ app for up-to-date lists of high- and low-FODMAP foods.

HOW DO FODMAPS TRIGGER SYMPTOMS?

We've just learned that FODMAPs are a large group of dietary sugars (short-chain carbohydrates) that can lead to an upset gut. The trouble begins when our small intestine fails to absorb these carbohydrates. The presence of FODMAPs causes water to be dragged into the small intestines, which can lead to diarrhea.

The malabsorbed sugars then travel on to our large intestine where they become "fast food" for our gut bacteria. FODMAPs provide these healthy bacteria with energy; however, as the gut bacteria feast, they rapidly ferment these short-chain carbohydrates. This produces large quantities of

gases (hydrogen, methane, and carbon dioxide). These gases are why FODMAPs cause flatulence and can lead to bloating and constipation.

This combination of excess water and gas production in the digestive tract causes our intestines to expand, making us bloated. This bloating distends our intestinal walls, irritating our highly sensitive nerve endings and triggering pain signals.

To combat these symptoms, the low-FODMAP diet works by reducing the overall FODMAPs consumed to a level our bodies can tolerate, helping to reduce diarrhea, flatulence, bloating and distention, abdominal pain, and constipation.

THREE PHASES OF THE LOW-FODMAP DIET

The low-FODMAP diet isn't for life; instead, it's a "teaching tool" to help you identify trigger foods. It's recommended that you undertake the diet with the help of a FODMAP-trained dietitian, who will help you break the low-FODMAP diet into three phases.

PHASE ONE: THE RESTRICTION PHASE

This phase of the low-FODMAP diet is all about reducing your FODMAP intake by removing high-FODMAP foods from your diet. The goal is to see if consuming fewer FODMAPs helps to significantly and consistently reduce your abdominal symptoms.

During this phase you will focus on eating low-FODMAP foods for two to six weeks to see if your symptoms settle. You have two options:

1. A *simplified low-FODMAP diet*, where you only remove foods that are very high in the FODMAPs that you eat on a regular basis. This option is a less restrictive approach and is appropriate if you experience only mild to moderate gastrointestinal symptoms or have a limited ability to restrict your diet.

2. A *strict low-FODMAP diet*, which involves removing all high-FODMAP foods from your diet. This approach is more restrictive and requires more effort and willpower. It's a good choice if you experience more severe symptoms.

It's important that you understand that the low-FODMAP diet isn't a magic cure for IBS; instead, our goal is to help you significantly reduce symptoms. The Monash University Low-FODMAP Diet™ app, certified low-FODMAP products, and the recipes in this cookbook are all fantastic resources for this stage of the diet.

PHASE TWO: THE RE-CHALLENGE PHASE

Once you know that reducing FODMAPs has helped you manage your symptoms, it's time to re-challenge high-FODMAP foods. If you are feeling good, then it's tempting to skip this phase altogether but FODMAPs contain important prebiotics. These prebiotics nourish gut bacteria and are important for long-term health. To protect your health, you need to figure out which FODMAPs you can reintroduce into your diet. You have two re-challenge options:

1. *Simplified re-challenge*: This is a simplified approach to testing FODMAPs. You will still test all the FODMAP groups but use a more simplified challenge schedule.
2. *Full re-challenge*: This version of the re-challenge phase takes eight to ten weeks. It comprehensively and systematically guides you through testing each of the FODMAP groups. During this phase you try specific foods that contain only one FODMAP group.

It's really important that during re-challenges you continue to eat low-FODMAP foods, so you can easily identify reactions when you eat the high-FODMAP food. This means that even if you don't experience gut symptoms from a challenge, you still need to remove that food from your diet and not reintroduce that FODMAP group until you have completed all the re-challenges. If you do experience gut symptoms, you should stop the

challenge and return to the low-FODMAP phase. Just remember that with each re-challenge test, you are assessing your tolerance to a FODMAP group, not the individual food.

A FODMAP-trained dietitian will help you determine which foods and at what doses are right for you to re-challenge with. For a more detailed overview and lots of re-challenge resources, go to alittlebityummy.com.

PHASE THREE: THE MODIFIED FODMAP DIET

In this phase you will build on your FODMAP re-challenge knowledge and find your food freedom. You should now have a good understanding of which FODMAP groups you can enjoy and how much you can eat. This means you can reintroduce back into your diet the FODMAPs you tolerated well, and figure out which combinations you can indulge in while keeping your symptoms settled.

Have fun relaxing your diet and remember to only limit the FODMAP groups you react to. It's also good to note that FODMAP intolerances can change over time, so go back and re-challenge FODMAP groups every now and then to see if your tolerance levels have changed.

FODMAP TIPS FOR SUCCESS

I understand that starting the low-FODMAP diet can be emotionally challenging. Setting up a good foundation for the diet before you start can make the journey easier:

1. Get the right support—the support and guidance of a FODMAP-trained dietitian can help you get your symptoms managed faster. Your dietitian can adjust the diet to suit your needs and suggest additional strategies that will complement your IBS toolbox.
2. Download the Monash University Low-FODMAP Diet™ app for up-to-date food

lists—this app is my bible and has been designed by Monash University, the lead researchers of the low-FODMAP diet. It contains up-to-date lists of low- and high-FODMAP foods as well as portion size info.

3. Take time to plan ahead—grab a cup of tea, this book, and your FODMAP app, and take some time to plan out your meals for each week. Don't forget to include some emergency snack ideas for when you get hungry. If you need more help, head over to alittlebityummy.com for more resources.

4. Find suitable products—stock your pantry with a range of low-FODMAP products to help make cooking fun. There are lots of ideas on pages 21, 22, and 29. Also check out the Monash University Low-FODMAP Diet™ app and the FODMAP Friendly app for certified low-FODMAP products.

5. Breathe! Don't try to be perfect—no one is perfect and it's likely that you will accidentally eat a high-FODMAP food during the first phase of the diet. That's okay! If you do experience symptoms, they should subside after a day or two. As the FODMAPs move out of your system, just continue eating low-FODMAP foods. Once you know that a low-FODMAP diet helps settle your gut, start re-challenging FODMAPs and find your food freedom.

UNDERSTANDING PORTION SIZES

Many people find that focusing on eating low-FODMAP foods is enough to gain good symptom relief. The goal of the low-FODMAP diet isn't to completely eliminate your symptoms, as a little bit of bloating and wind is normal and healthy. However, a low-FODMAP diet is a fairly fluid concept. Many foods that are low FODMAP at a smaller serving become high FODMAP at a larger serving size.

A low-FODMAP serving is a serving of food that falls under the FODMAP cut-off levels that might trigger symptoms. The low-FODMAP diet is not a no-FODMAP diet, which means even low-FODMAP foods can still contain some FODMAPs.

Here are some examples:

- Rolled oats are low FODMAP in ½-cup servings but larger servings can contain moderate amounts of oligosaccharides.
- Sweet potato is a high-FODMAP food that can be enjoyed in ½-cup low-FODMAP servings, but larger servings are high in mannitol.
- Canned tomatoes are low-FODMAP in 3-ounce (90g) servings but at 4 ounces (115g) contain moderate amounts of excess fructose.

(Source: Monash University Low-FODMAP Diet™ app)

These foods can all be enjoyed in the first phase of the diet—just watch your portion sizes! You can find detailed information on each low-FODMAP food in the Food Guide of the Monash University Low FODMAP Diet™ app.

HOW TO AVOID FODMAP STACKING

You might be wondering how you can safely combine foods if low-FODMAP foods still contain FODMAPs. The FODMAP cut-off levels are conservative; this means you can comfortably combine multiple low-FODMAP portion sizes of different foods in a meal.

If you want to increase your serving size of a low-FODMAP food, check for FODMAP notes in the Monash University Low FODMAP Diet™ app first. You might be pleasantly surprised to find you can eat the food freely! If a couple of foods in your meal contain a warning for the same FODMAP group, then you might find that having a whole serving of one food and a half serving of another food is a better option for you.

You can eat the same food several times in one day, just leave three to four hours between each serving.

LOW-FODMAP FRUIT AND PORTION SIZES

If you are a fruit lover, then you might need to ration your fruit over the course of your day. It is recommended that you enjoy one serving of low-FODMAP fruit per meal and leave three hours between each serving.

Many low-FODMAP smoothie recipes can be FODMAP bombs as they simply contain too many servings of fruit. I love smoothies, so I have created some delicious low-FODMAP options on page 40 that keep to low-FODMAP serving size guidelines.

LOOKING AFTER YOUR GUT HEALTH

In the initial phase of the low-FODMAP diet, it's important that you protect your gut health until you can add back in some high-FODMAP foods.

High-FODMAP foods contain prebiotics, which nourish our good gut bugs and keep our digestive system healthy. When we remove these foods, we also reduce the food our gut bugs get to eat. We don't know the long-term effect of this yet, but we do know that limiting food to our gut bugs has a significant impact on our gut microbiome by reducing the numbers and diversity of our healthy gut bacteria.

During the initial phase of the low-FODMAP diet, you can help nourish your healthy gut bugs by eating low-FODMAP foods that contain prebiotic fibers and low-FODMAP servings of high-FODMAP foods. Try to include a few of the foods below in your meals.

- Fruits: Firm banana, pomegranate seeds,* rambutan,* currants/raisins/cranberries,* kiwifruit, rhubarb
- Vegetables: Savoy cabbage,* red cabbage, common cabbage, corn,* fennel bulb,* snow peas,* yuca,* taro*
- Grains: Rolled oats, puffed amaranth,* buckwheat kernels,* wheat bran,* quinoa
- Pasta: Cooked spelt or wheat pasta*
- Bread: Spelt or wheat sourdough bread*
- Pulses: Canned lentils,* canned chickpeas,* canned butter beans,* boiled lima beans,* boiled mung beans*
- Nuts: Small handful of almonds* or hazelnuts*

*These foods have small low-FODMAP servings. Check the Monash University Low FODMAP Diet™ app for more information and avoid large servings as they do become high FODMAP.

After a few weeks on the low-FODMAP diet, make sure you move into the re-challenge phase so you can work out which high-FODMAP foods to add back into your diet. This will help you increase your prebiotic intake and protect your gut health in the long run.

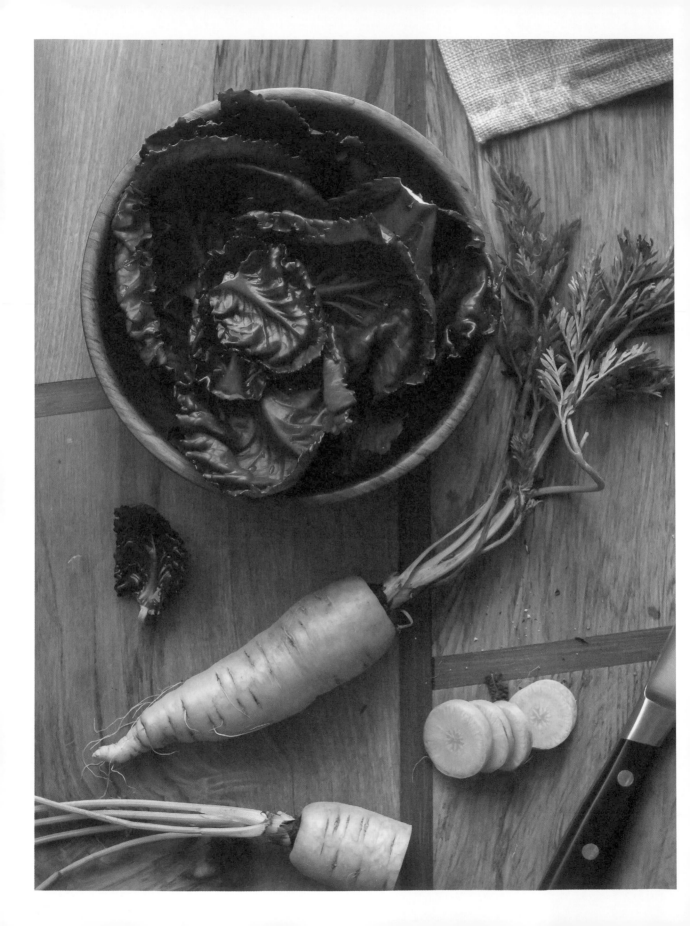

Filling Your Fridge
LOW-FODMAP SEASONAL PRODUCE

Choosing seasonal produce is a great way to budget and enjoy veggies all year-round! Just check the Monash University Low FODMAP Diet™ app for serving size guidelines.

SPRING

Blueberries,* broccoli, common cabbage, endive, lettuce, mustard greens, radicchio, radishes, raspberries,* red cabbage, strawberries, Swiss chard, zucchini.*

SUMMER

Bell peppers, blueberries,* broccoli, cherry tomatoes, corn (limit to 3 tablespoons of kernels), cucumber, eggplant, green beans, kabocha squash/Japanese pumpkin, leeks (only use the green leaves), lettuce, strawberries, Swiss chard, tomatoes, zucchini.*

AUTUMN

Bell peppers, cherry tomatoes, collard greens, common cabbage, corn (limit to 3 tablespoons of kernels), cucumber, eggplant, endive, green beans, kabocha squash/Japanese pumpkin, kiwifruit, leeks (only use the green leaves), lettuce, limes, mandarins, parsnips, red cabbage, rutabaga, spaghetti squash, tomatoes, turnips, zucchini.*

WINTER

Collard greens, common cabbage, endive, kabocha squash/Japanese pumpkin, kiwifruit, leeks (only use the green leaves), lemons, limes, mandarins, mustard greens, oranges, parsnips, radicchio, radishes, red cabbage, rutabaga, spaghetti squash, turnips.

ALL YEAR-ROUND

Arugula, bananas, bok choy, carrots, frozen green beans, grapes, kale, potatoes, rhubarb, watercress.

*Small servings are low FODMAP—check the Monash University Low FODMAP Diet app for guidelines

Stocking Your Pantry

The low-FODMAP diet does require you to get creative in the kitchen! Below are some of my favorite low-FODMAP ingredients to help you stock your pantry and to create meals that your whole family will love. Check the Monash University Low FODMAP Diet™ app for serving sizes.

HERBS AND SPICES

Chile powder/crushed red pepper*
Chinese five spice*
Curry powder*
Dried basil
Dried oregano
Dried sage
Dried thyme
Ground coriander
Ground cumin
Mustard seeds
Paprika
Saffron
Turmeric

OILS

Garlic-infused oil
Neutral oil (canola, grapeseed, safflower, sunflower)
Olive oil
Sesame oil

CEREALS AND GRAINS

Corn chips*
Corn starch
Corn tortillas
Gluten-free all-purpose flour*
Gluten-free bread*
Gluten-free pasta*
Millet
Quinoa
Rice (white or brown)
Rice noodles

SWEETENERS

Brown sugar
Molasses**
Pure maple syrup
Rice malt syrup
White/granulated sugar

CONDIMENTS

Balsamic vinegar**
Crushed or pureed ginger
Fish sauce
Low-FODMAP stock (chicken or vegetable)
Mayonnaise
Mustard*
Oyster sauce**
Rice wine vinegar
Red wine vinegar
Soy sauce
Worcestershire sauce

LEGUMES

Canned chickpeas**
Canned lentils**

CANNED VEGETABLES

Beets
Champignon mushrooms

*Check for added high-FODMAP ingredients
**Small servings are low-FODMAP—check the Monash app for guidelines

LABEL-READING SHOPPING GUIDE

High-FODMAP ingredients like to hide in processed products. These shopping guides can help you navigate the supermarket minefield and make shopping easier. Additional information on ingredients, and more extensive lists, can be found in the Monash University Low FODMAP Diet™ and FODMAP Friendly apps.

HIGH-FODMAP FLOURS	LOW-FODMAP ALTERNATIVES
Almond meal (more than ¼ cup per serving), amaranth flour, barley flour, coconut flour, einkorn flour, emmer flour, gram/besan/chickpea flour, khorasan (kamut) flour, lentil flour, lupin flour, rye flour, soy flour, spelt flour (unless it is sifted), wheat flour	Arrowroot flour, buckwheat flour, corn starch, green banana flour, maize flour, millet flour, potato starch, quinoa flour, rice flour, sorghum flour, tapioca starch, teff flour. FODMAP-certified breads Gluten-free flour and gluten-free bread (check for high-FODMAP flours and added high-FODMAP ingredients) Spelt sourdough bread Wheat sourdough bread
Common sources: Breads, pastries, and baked goods	**Notes**: If the wheat, rye, or barley is listed after the third ingredient in an ingredient list, then small amounts of the product may be low FODMAP. The same is true with soy or coconut flour if it is not the predominant flour in the product.
HIGH-FODMAP DAIRY PRODUCTS AND DAIRY ALTERNATIVES	**LOW-FODMAP ALTERNATIVES**
Dairy-based ingredients: Buttermilk, condensed milk, cow's milk, custard, evaporated milk, goat's milk, ice cream, lactose, milk curds, milk solids, sour cream, whey protein concentrate, yogurt Dairy alternatives: Coconut milk with inulin, oat milk, soy milk made with whole or hulled soy beans	Butter, goat's yogurt, lactose-free custard, lactose-free milk, lactose-free sour cream, lactose-free yogurt, most hard cheeses (e.g. Cheddar, Colby, Harvarti, mozzarella, Pecorino, Swiss), whey protein isolate. Almond milk, canned coconut milk,* coconut yogurt, hemp milk, macadamia milk, quinoa milk, rice milk,* soy milk made from soy protein, UHT coconut milk* *Check the Monash University Low FODMAP Diet™ app for serving size info
Common sources: Ice cream, milk products, protein powders, yogurt	**Notes**: Check low-FODMAP alternatives for added high-FODMAP ingredients like fructose, high-fructose corn syrup, high-FODMAP fruit juices, inulin (chicory root fiber)

HIGH-FODMAP SWEETENERS	LOW-FODMAP ALTERNATIVES
Agave syrup, apple juice, apple puree, crystalline fructose, date puree, fructose, fructo-oligosaccharides (FOS), fructose-glucose syrup, fruit concentrate, fruit juice, fruit sugar, high-fructose corn syrup, honey, isoglucose, molasses,** pear juice, yacon syrup Sweeteners: Isomalt, maltitol, mannitol, sorbitol, xylitol **These foods have small low-FODMAP servings. Check the Monash University Low FODMAP Diet™ app for more information	Beet sugar, brown sugar, confectioners' sugar, corn syrup, dextrose, glucose syrup, palm sugar, pure maple syrup, rice malt syrup, stevia, superfine sugar, table syrup, white sugar
Common sources: Baked goods, breads, breakfast cereals, gluten-free products, jams, lactose-free or coconut yogurts, protein powders, soft drinks, sports drinks	

HIGH-FODMAP SOURCES OF ONION AND GARLIC	LOW-FODMAP ALTERNATIVES
Chicken salt, dehydrated vegetables, garlic, preprepared spice mixes (e.g. Moroccan or Mexican)	All fresh and dried herbs Asafoetida powder Dried spices (no added onion or garlic) Garlic-infused oil
Common sources: Commercial sauces and dressings, flavored rice crackers and potato chips, savory products, stock/broth, soups	

OTHER PROBLEMATIC INGREDIENTS	COMMON LOW-FODMAP INGREDIENTS
Chicory root extract, chicory root fiber, dietary fiber, inulin	Acidity regulators, anti-caking agents, antifoaming agents, antioxidants, barley malt extract (small servings), caramel color, carrageenan, cellulose, colors, colorings and color fixatives, enzymes, flavor enhancers, foaming agents, fruit flavors/extracts, guar gum, locust bean gum, pectins, preservatives, psyllium, raising agents (baking powder or baking soda), rice/oat bran, soy lecithin, soy sauce, thickeners, xanthan gum
Common sources: Baked goods, coconut yogurt, dairy-free alternatives, gluten-free bread, lactose-free dairy products, premade sauces or dressings, rice crackers	

FODMAP AND GLUTEN-FREE BUYING TIPS

These buying tips will help you avoid sneaky FODMAPs in common recipe ingredients. Just remember that the low-FODMAP diet isn't a gluten-free diet, and we remove large servings of wheat, rye, and barley due to the fructans (oligosaccharides), not the gluten. I have provided additional gluten-free tips for those of you who are also managing celiac disease and need a strict gluten-free diet.

FODMAP BUYING TIPS

INGREDIENT	BUYING TIP
Bacon	Check that the bacon hasn't been cured with honey.
Canned pineapple in syrup	If possible choose canned pineapple in syrup sweetened with sugar rather than high-fructose corn syrup or pear juice. Rinse well before using.
Chile powder/flakes	Choose pure chile powder/crushed red pepper that does not contain any onion or garlic powder.
Chile puree	Choose plain pureed chile. Avoid brands that contain garlic.
Chinese five spice	Avoid Chinese five spice powders that contain garlic.
Crushed ginger	Choose plain crushed or pureed ginger.
Curry powder	Avoid brands that include garlic or onion powder.
Dried cranberries	Avoid dried cranberries that have been sweetened with apple juice or high-fructose corn syrup.
Garlic-infused oil	Garlic-infused oil is a low-FODMAP alternative to garlic. It contains the flavor but not the FODMAPs. Look for an infused oil that doesn't contain garlic pieces.
Gluten-free all-purpose or self-rising flour	Choose a gluten-free flour mix that doesn't contain amaranth flour, chickpea/besan flour, coconut flour, lentil flour, or soy flour.
Gluten-free cornflakes	Avoid cornflakes sweetened with apple or pear juice, fruit juice, honey, or high-fructose corn syrup.
Gluten-free pasta	Avoid gluten-free pastas that include amaranth flour, inulin, lupin flour, or soy flour.
Lactose-free yogurt or coconut yogurt	Check for fruit juice, fructose, high-FODMAP fruits, high-fructose corn syrup, and inulin.

INGREDIENT	BUYING TIP
Low-FODMAP bread/gluten-free bread/gluten-free breadcrumbs	Check for high-FODMAP flours and added high-FODMAP ingredients such as fruit juice, high-fructose corn syrup, honey, and inulin. Check your FODMAP app for certified brands.
Low-FODMAP chicken or vegetable bouillon powder	Watch out for onion or garlic powder. Check your FODMAP app for certified brands.
Low-FODMAP chicken or vegetable stock	Avoid brands that contain onion or garlic, or make your own chicken stock as on page 212.
Low-FODMAP milk	See opposite for low-FODMAP milk options.
Mustard (wholegrain or Dijon)	Check that the mustard does not contain any garlic or onion.
Plant-based milks including almond, coconut, rice and soy protein milk	Check that the milk does not contain chicory root, fructose, high-fructose corn syrup, or inulin.
Sliced ham	Check the ham doesn't include garlic, honey, or onion powder. Or use leftover ham (see page 192).
Soy sauce	This sauce is fermented and is low FODMAP in small servings, despite often containing wheat. It is not necessary to buy gluten-free soy sauce.
Vegan cheese	Avoid brands that contain cashews, garlic, or onion.
Whole chicken	Whole chickens can be packaged in broth or seasoned. Check that these don't include onion or garlic.
Worcestershire sauce	This sauce is fermented and is low FODMAP in small servings despite often containing onion or garlic.

GLUTEN-FREE BUYING TIPS

If you have celiac disease, please check all dried herbs, dried fruit, nuts, seeds, and spices for trace gluten.

Also choose gluten-free options for soy sauce, low-FODMAP chicken stock, Worcestershire sauce, corn starch, confectioners' sugar, baking powder, and baking soda. You can often find guar gum and xanthan gum in the gluten-free area of the supermarket, or at your local health food store. Check other processed foods for trace gluten.

HOW TO CHOOSE A LOW-FODMAP MILK

Choosing a low-FODMAP milk option is an essential part of building your pantry and creating delicious low-FODMAP meals. Regular cow's milk is considered high FODMAP as it contains lactose, but luckily there are lots of suitable alternatives.

LOW-FODMAP MILK OPTIONS

Low-FODMAP milk options include almond milk, canned coconut milk,* hemp milk, lactose-free milk, macadamia milk, rice milk,* soy milk (made from soy protein), UHT coconut milk,* and unsweetened quinoa milk.
*These milks have low-FODMAP servings, but your portion size needs to be limited. Check the Monash University Low FODMAP Diet™ app for more information.

NUTRITION TIPS

Many dairy-free milks are a poor source of protein and do not naturally contain suitable amounts of calcium or other micronutrients. If you are using an alternative milk, make sure it has been fortified with calcium.
- Check the nutrition panel and look for at least 120mg of calcium per 100ml.
- For children or those with high energy needs, look for products with around 3g protein/100ml and 3g fat/100ml.

WATCH OUT FOR SNEAKY FODMAPS

Many milk substitutes have added high-FODMAP ingredients such as agave syrup, chicory root extract, fructose, high-fructose corn syrup, honey, inulin, or molasses. Check your milk substitute for high-FODMAP ingredients before you buy.

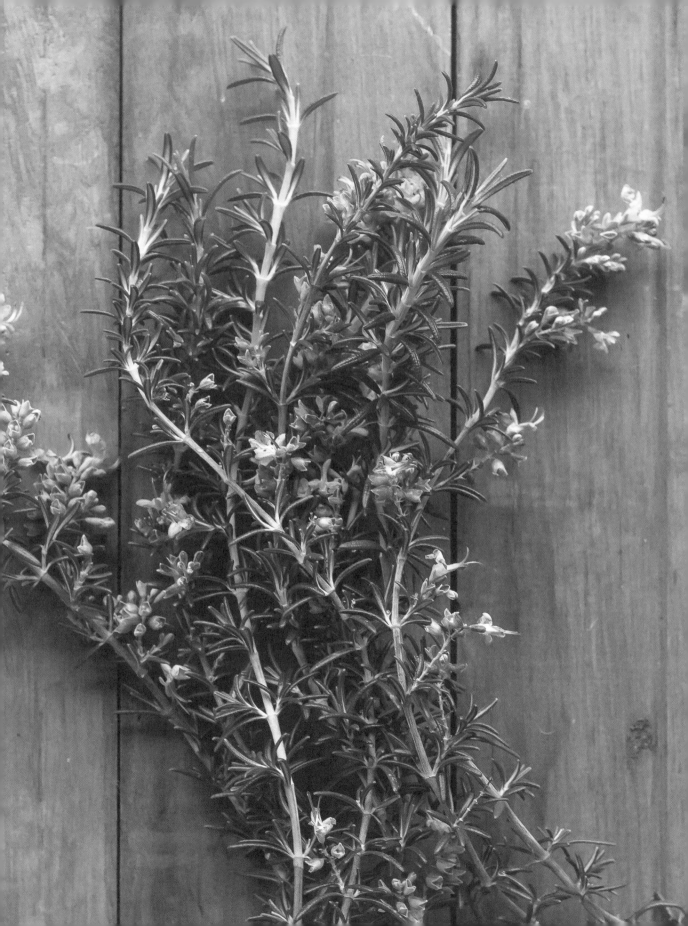

Recapturing Flavor

EASY LOW-FODMAP SWAPS

Re-creating family favorites and boosting the flavor of your low-FODMAP meals is easy with these simple low-FODMAP swaps.

GARLIC

- Garlic-infused oil
- Asafoetida powder

Cooking tip: For a cooked meal (such as spaghetti Bolognese), try using 1 tablespoon of garlic-infused oil for 4 servings. For raw dishes (such as aïoli), start with a few drops. Or try frying a small pinch of asafoetida powder in cooking oil before adding other ingredients.

ONION

- Green leaves of leeks or scallions
- Fresh or dried chives

Cooking tip: Replace 1 onion with about 1 cup of diced green leek leaves or scallion tips. If using scallion tips or chives, mix into the meal in the last 5 minutes of cooking.

HONEY

- Pure maple syrup
- Brown sugar
- Rice malt syrup

Cooking tip: For most recipes you can usually replace the honey with an equal quantity of the low-FODMAP alternative.

BREAD OR MILK

- Gluten-free bread or spelt/wheat sourdough
- Lactose-free milk or low-FODMAP milk alternative (see page 25).

Cooking tip: Replace in 1:1 ratios. Check low-FODMAP alternatives for high-FODMAP ingredients (see Label-Reading Shopping Guide, page 23).

FLAVOR-BOOSTING TIPS

Learning to cook low-FODMAP style encourages you to get creative in the kitchen. I love using these easy tricks to boost the flavors in my recipes.

BRIGHTEN FLAVORS BY ADDING AN ACID

Try adding a squeeze of lemon juice or a few drops of vinegar at the end of cooking. The sourness of the acid will brighten the other flavors.

SEASON WITH SALT AND PEPPER

Don't be afraid to add a few grinds of salt and pepper every time you add a batch of ingredients to the pan. This will help enhance the flavor.

EMBRACE FRESH HERBS AND SPICES

Most herbs and spices are low FODMAP so you can add generous amounts to your meal. Try adding a handful of fresh herbs to your next salad, risotto, or stir-fry.

BALANCE SWEETNESS AND SPICE

Everyone has different taste preferences. Don't be afraid to add some spice by using crushed red pepper or fresh chile powder. Or add a touch of sweetness with some maple syrup, rice malt syrup, or brown sugar.

ADD A SPLASH OF STOCK OR WINE

Boost the flavor of your meal by adding a splash of low-FODMAP stock or wine.

ALLERGY ICONS

I understand how challenging it can be trying to eat low FODMAP when you have other food intolerances. This cookbook is allergy friendly, so you can create meals that love you back.

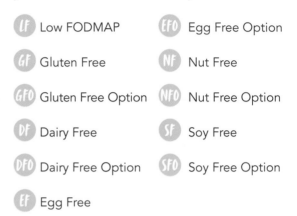

LF Low FODMAP

GF Gluten Free

GFO Gluten Free Option

DF Dairy Free

DFO Dairy Free Option

EF Egg Free

EFO Egg Free Option

NF Nut Free

NFO Nut Free Option

SF Soy Free

SFO Soy Free Option

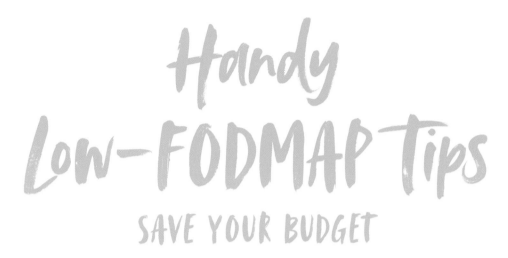

Handy Low-FODMAP Tips

SAVE YOUR BUDGET

Shopping on the low-FODMAP diet can be expensive. These 11 budget-saving tips will make sure your grocery list doesn't break the bank.

1. Plan your meals and write a shopping list. This will help stop you impulse buying and walking aimlessly around the supermarket.
2. Check out independent grocery stores, Asian supermarkets, and butchers in your area. They often have lower prices and good-quality produce.
3. Cook extra for dinner and take leftovers for lunch. It is much cheaper to cook in bulk and it reduces the amount of meal-prep work you need to do each week.
4. Re-grow your scallions and leeks. In the low-FODMAP diet we can only use the green leaves of both scallions and leeks. Place the scallion bulbs and leek bulbs in glasses of water on your window sill. Let them reshoot and then plant them in the garden.
5. Use frozen vegetables and berries. Check the frozen aisle for low-FODMAP options such as green beans, broccoli, carrots, strawberries, raspberries, and blueberries.
6. Invest in a variety of dried herbs or grow your own fresh herbs.
7. Focus on using potatoes, rice, and rice noodles as fillers in your meals. Keep gluten-free pasta as an occasional treat.
8. Save money on meat. Try using canned fish, such as tuna and salmon, lean ground meat, shellfish, eggs, and firm tofu as cheap and versatile protein sources.
9. Make your own lactose-free milk. You can make your own by adding lactase drops to standard cow's milk (the lactase enzymes digest the lactose, making it low FODMAP). These are available from pharmacies, or you can buy them online.
10. Make your own gluten-free baking at home.
11. Carry a water bottle instead of buying bottled drinks.

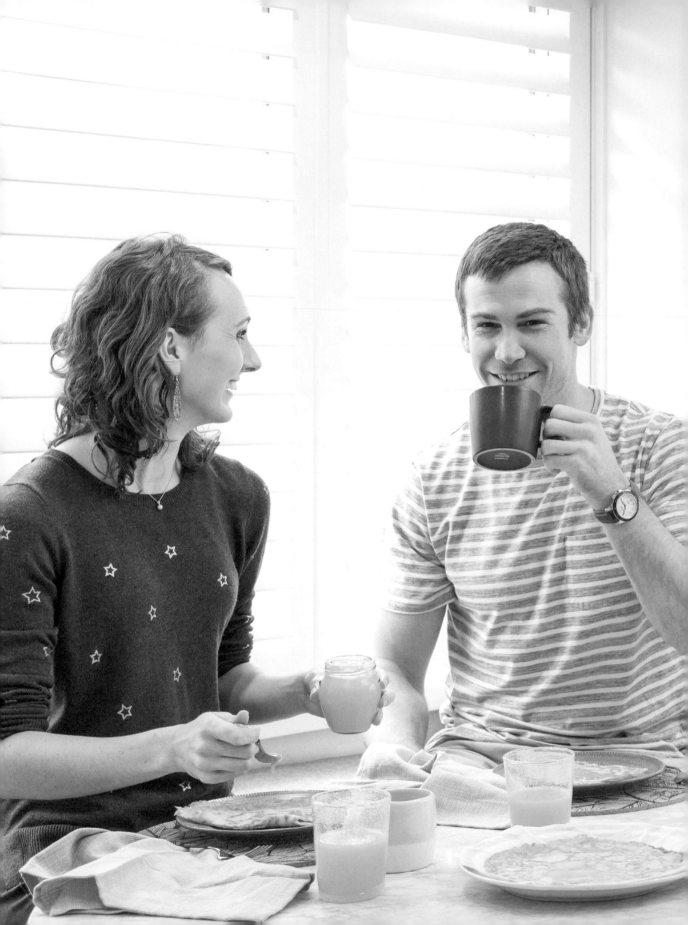

BREAKFAST

Nourish your body and soul with
a delicious low-FODMAP breakfast!

Crêpes with Lemon Curd & Passionfruit

PREP TIME: 5 minutes COOK TIME: 35 minutes
MAKES: 10 crêpes (serves 4–5)

LF · GF · DFO · NF · SF

1 cup (140g) gluten-free all-purpose
   flour*
2 eggs
2 tablespoons dairy-free spread or
   butter, melted
½ cup (125ml) low-FODMAP milk*
¾ cup (185ml) water
½ teaspoon salt
Olive oil or butter, for cooking
5 tablespoons Lemon Curd (see recipe
   on page 216; 1 tablespoon per
   serving)
4 passionfruit
Confectioners' sugar (GF if needed),
   for dusting

Growing up, crêpes were always my favorite holiday treat.
I now love combining crêpes with one of my favorite flavor
combos—lemon curd and passionfruit—to achieve the perfect
balance between sweet and tart.

1 In a blender, combine the flour, eggs, dairy-free spread or
butter, milk, water, and salt until smooth (you can make the
batter up to a day before and keep it in the fridge). Chill in the
fridge for 30 minutes. Test the batter: it should pour smoothly
out of a cup. If it "plops" instead, thin the batter with a little
more water.

2 Heat a 12-inch nonstick frying pan over low to medium
heat and coat lightly with olive oil or butter. Add ¼ cup of
batter and swirl until it completely covers the bottom of
the pan. Cook the crêpe for about 2 minutes, then peek
underneath—if the crêpe is golden brown, it's time to flip and
cook for another minute.

3 Add more olive oil or butter and repeat with the remaining
crêpe batter.

4 Top each crêpe with a drizzle of lemon curd, a spoonful of
passionfruit pulp, and a dusting of confectioners' sugar.

TIPS
*Check buying tips (see pages
25–27).

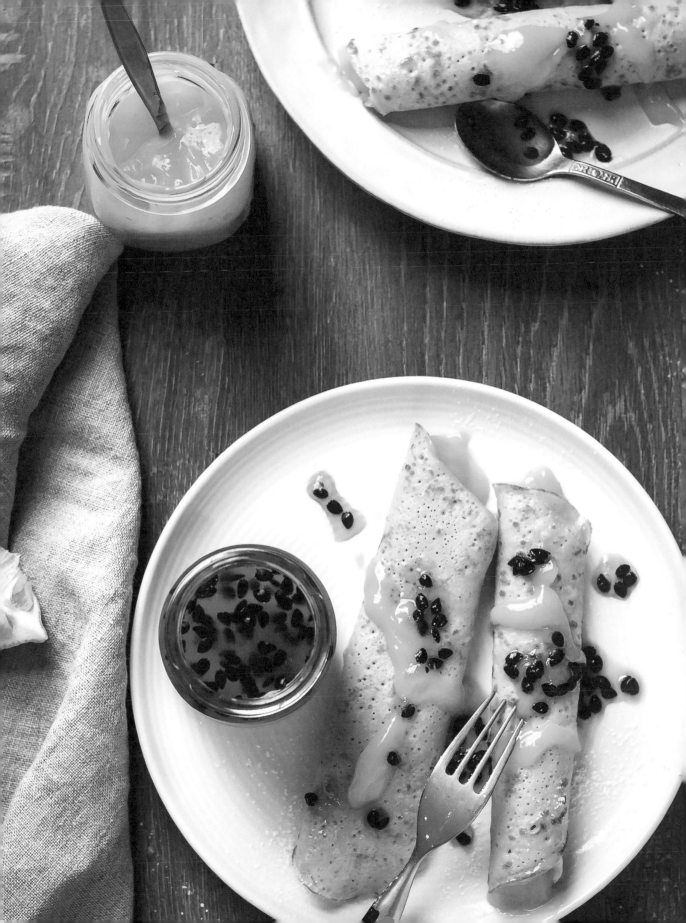

Coconut Chia Rice Pudding with Stewed Rhubarb & Strawberries

PREP TIME: 10 minutes **COOK TIME:** 1½ hours
SERVES: 4

LF GF DFO NF EF SF

COCONUT CHIA RICE PUDDING

½ cup short-grain rice
1½ tablespoons chia seeds
2 cups (500ml) coconut milk (UHT)*
3 cups (750ml) low-FODMAP milk*
¼ cup (60ml) water
½ teaspoon ground cinnamon
1 tablespoon pure maple syrup
    (optional)

STEWED RHUBARB & STRAWBERRIES

2 cups (7oz/200g) chopped rhubarb,
    washed and cut into small pieces
2 cups (10oz/280g) fresh or frozen
    strawberries
⅓ cup (85ml) water
Drizzle of pure maple syrup (optional)
Handful of toasted pumpkin seeds, to
    serve (optional)

This rice pudding makes a delicious hot breakfast or a yummy dessert. I love topping mine with stewed rhubarb and strawberries.

1 Preheat oven to 325°F. Place the rice, chia seeds, coconut milk, milk, water, and cinnamon in a large ovenproof dish. Mix well. Place in the oven, uncovered.

2 Cook for 1½ hours, stirring every 20–30 minutes to break up the skin that forms. Remove once the rice is thick and creamy.

3 Leave to cool for a few minutes, then taste. Stir in the maple syrup, if desired.

4 While the rice pudding cooks, make the stewed fruit. Place the rhubarb and strawberries in a medium saucepan. Add the water and cover with a lid. Place over medium heat for 6–8 minutes, until the fruit softens and starts to collapse as it is stirred. Add more maple syrup to taste, if needed.

5 Serve the rice pudding with the stewed rhubarb and strawberries. Sprinkle with toasted pumpkin seeds, if desired.

TIPS

As the rice pudding cools, it will become quite solid. That's okay, as it will soften when you reheat it. Just add an extra splash of milk to loosen the mixture before popping it into the microwave. Store in the fridge for up to 4 days.

*Check buying tips (see page 27).

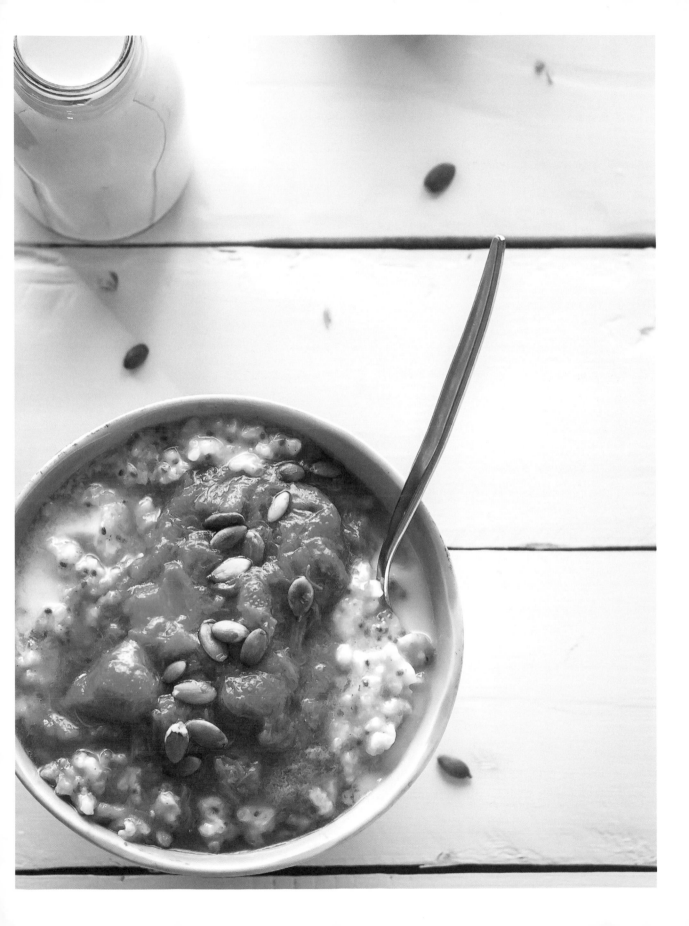

Poached Eggs with Lemon Hollandaise Sauce

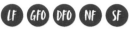

PREP TIME: 10 minutes **COOK TIME**: 10 minutes
SERVES: 2

1 tablespoon white vinegar

4 eggs

Buttered low-FODMAP or gluten-free toast,* to serve

Handful of mixed lettuce leaves, to serve

A few grinds of salt and pepper

LEMON HOLLANDAISE SAUCE

1½ tablespoons lemon juice

2 egg yolks

⅛ teaspoon white sugar

Pinch of rock salt

Black pepper, to taste

2 tablespoons dairy-free spread or butter

This is my idea of a perfect lazy Sunday breakfast!

1 Fill a deep frying pan with about 1¼ inches of water and add the vinegar. Bring the water to a rolling boil, then turn down to a gentle simmer.

2 Take an egg and crack it into a small sieve (this removes any loose egg white and gives you a pretty poached egg), then carefully pour it into a small bowl.

3 Stir the water until it swirls and carefully pour the whole egg into the pan. Repeat for each egg. Cook each egg for about 2 minutes for a soft egg or 4 minutes for a firmer egg, then scoop out and place on a paper towel to drain.

4 Make the hollandaise sauce while the eggs cook. Whisk the lemon juice, egg yolks, sugar, salt, and black pepper together in a small bowl until smooth. Melt the dairy-free spread or butter in the microwave and slowly whisk into the mixture.

5 Heat the hollandaise sauce in the microwave for 15 seconds, whisk, and then heat in 10-second bursts (you might need to do this four or five times), whisking each time to remove the skin that forms on the sides of the bowl. Repeat until thick.

6 Serve the poached eggs on buttered toast with mixed lettuce leaves. Drizzle with hollandaise sauce and season with salt and pepper to taste.

TIPS

*Check buying tips (see page 26).

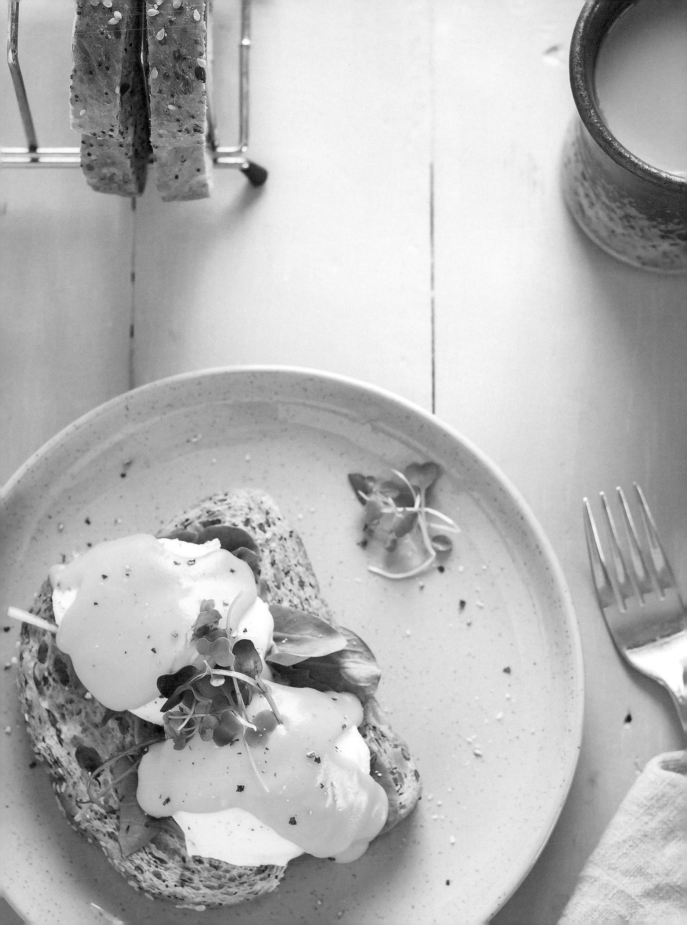

Smoothie Time

EACH SMOOTHIE SERVES: 1
PREP TIME: 5 minutes

(LF) (GFO) (DFO) (EF) (NF) (SF)

Smoothies can often be FODMAP bombs . . . so I have created some delicious low-FODMAP options that include the equivalent of only one serving of fruit. Enjoy!

1 Place all the ingredients for your chosen smoothie in a blender and blitz until smooth. If at any point the smoothie becomes too thick, add a splash of cold water.

STRAWBERRY SMOOTHIE

½ cup (125ml) low-FODMAP milk*

1 cup (5oz/140g) fresh or frozen strawberries, chopped

¼ cup (60ml) lactose-free yogurt or coconut yogurt*

1 teaspoon chia seeds (optional)

½ tablespoon pure maple syrup

1 teaspoon lemon juice

¼ teaspoon vanilla essence

6 ice cubes (if using fresh strawberries)

PINEAPPLE SMOOTHIE

2½ ounces (70g) fresh pineapple, cut into pieces and frozen

1 ounce (30g) firm banana (no brown spots), cut into pieces and frozen

¼ cup (60ml) coconut yogurt*

½ teaspoon vanilla essence

1 cup (250ml) low-FODMAP milk*

1 teaspoon pure maple syrup (optional)

4 ice cubes

BANANA CHOCOLATE SMOOTHIE

1 small (2½oz/80g) firm banana (no brown spots), cut into pieces and frozen

1 cup (250ml) low-FODMAP milk*

1 tablespoon cocoa powder (GF if needed)

½ teaspoon vanilla essence

2 teaspoons pure maple syrup

⅛ teaspoon ground cinnamon (optional)

5 ice cubes

BLUEBERRY SMOOTHIE

½ cup (125ml) low-FODMAP milk*

¼ cup (60ml) lactose-free yogurt or coconut yogurt*

20 fresh or frozen blueberries

6 ice cubes

1 ounce (30g) firm banana (no brown spots), cut into pieces and frozen

1 teaspoon chia seeds (optional)

½ tablespoon pure maple syrup (optional)

1 teaspoon lemon juice

TIPS
*Check buying tips (see pages 25–27).

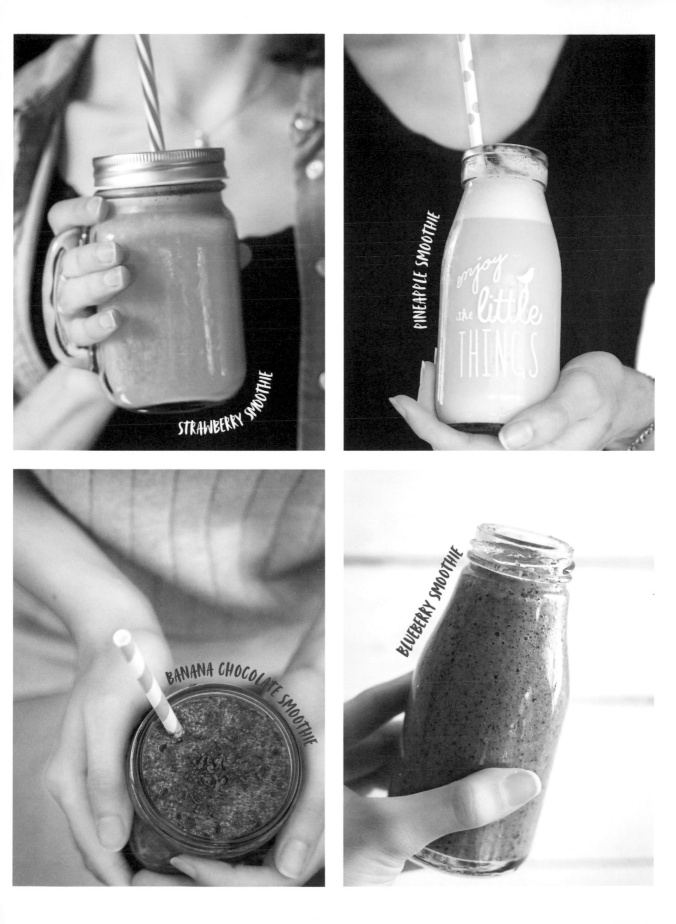

STRAWBERRY SMOOTHIE

PINEAPPLE SMOOTHIE

BANANA CHOCOLATE SMOOTHIE

BLUEBERRY SMOOTHIE

Crunchy Toasted Granola

PREP TIME: 5 minutes COOK TIME: 30 minutes
SERVES: 6 (½ cup per serving)

LF GFO DF NFO EF SF

2 tablespoons pure maple syrup

2 tablespoons brown sugar

4 tablespoons olive oil

¼ cup pecans or pumpkin seeds

¼ cup raw sunflower seeds

½ cup dried banana chips

6 tablespoons dried cranberries*

3 cups rolled oats

½ cup coconut chips or dried
    shredded coconut

¼ cup sesame seeds

1 teaspoon ground cinnamon

I developed this recipe for my best friend, who is a granola lover and on the low-FODMAP diet. She is super busy so I made sure this recipe would be quick and easy to fit into her schedule.

1 Preheat oven to 250°F.

2 Melt the maple syrup, brown sugar, and oil in the microwave in 20-second bursts until the sugar has dissolved.

3 Roughly chop the pecans or pumpkin seeds, sunflower seeds, banana chips, and cranberries. Set aside the cranberries and banana chips.

4 In a large bowl, mix together the rolled oats, pecans or pumpkin seeds, sunflower seeds, coconut chips, sesame seeds, cinnamon, and the sugar syrup.

5 Line a large baking sheet with parchment paper and evenly spread the granola over it.

6 Toast the granola in the oven for 25–30 minutes, stirring every 10 minutes until golden. Remove from the oven and mix in the cranberries and banana chips. Cool completely before transferring to an airtight container or glass jar.

7 Enjoy in ½-cup servings. If you are still feeling hungry, increase the serving size to ¾ cup.

TIPS

Please note this recipe is not gluten free. To make this recipe gluten free, swap the oats for a mixture of your favorite cereals. Gluten-free cornflakes, puffed quinoa or millet, and buckwheat or quinoa flakes should work well.

*Check buying tips (see page 25).

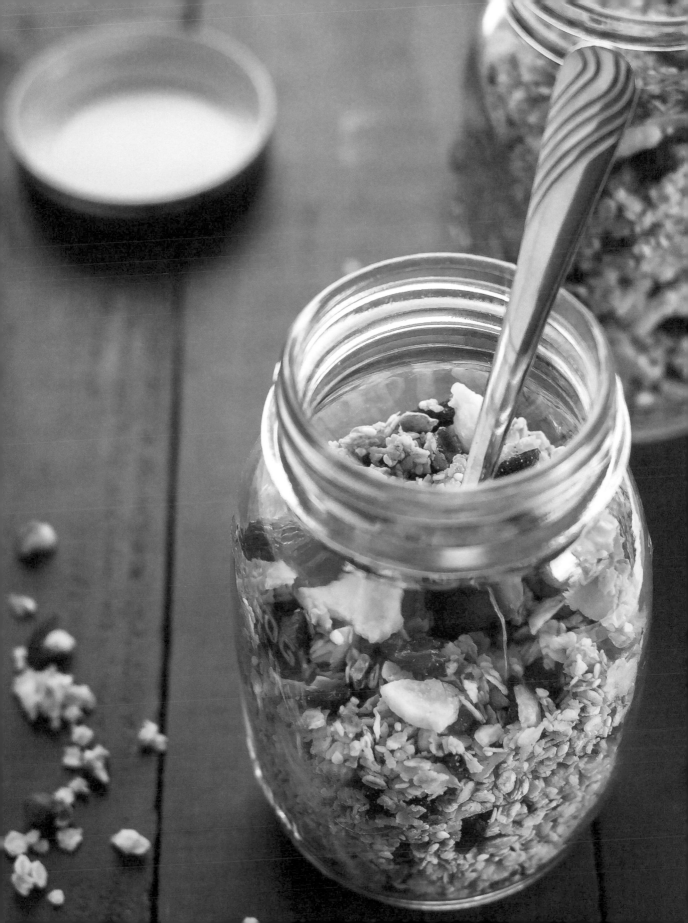

Tasty-Up Your Toast!

Banish boring breakfasts with these quick and easy low-FODMAP toast ideas.

BASIL PESTO WITH CHERRY TOMATOES ON TOAST
PREP TIME: 2 minutes **SERVES**: 1

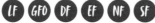

1 slice low-FODMAP or gluten-free bread*
1 tablespoon Easy Basil Pesto (see recipe on page 215)
5 cherry tomatoes, halved or quartered
A few fresh basil leaves, to serve (optional)
Black pepper, to taste

1 Toast the bread, spread with basil pesto, and top with cherry tomatoes. Garnish with basil leaves, if using.

2 Season with a few grinds of black pepper.

SMOKED SALMON & CHIVE DIP ON TOAST
PREP TIME: 4 minutes **SERVES**: 1

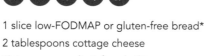

1 slice low-FODMAP or gluten-free bread*
2 tablespoons cottage cheese
¼ teaspoon garlic-infused oil*
½ teaspoon dried chives
¾ ounce (20g) plain smoked salmon
Fresh dill, to serve

1 Toast the bread. Mix the cottage cheese, oil, and chives together.

2 Spread the creamy chive dip on the toast and top with smoked salmon. Garnish with dill.

TIPS
*Check buying tips (see page 26).

AVOCADO & POACHED EGG ON TOAST
PREP TIME: 5 minutes **COOK TIME**: 5 minutes
SERVES: 1

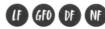

1 egg
2 tablespoons avocado
1 tablespoon mayonnaise
½ teaspoon lemon juice
Black pepper, to taste
1 slice low-FODMAP or gluten-free bread*
Fresh alfalfa sprouts, to serve (optional)

1 Poach the egg (see instructions on page 38). Mash together the avocado, mayonnaise, and lemon juice. Season well with black pepper. Toast the bread.

2 Spread the avocado mixture on the toast and top with the poached egg. Garnish with alfalfa sprouts, if using.

NUTTY BANANA TOAST
PREP TIME: 4 minutes **SERVES**: 1

1 slice low-FODMAP or gluten-free bread*
1 tablespoon peanut butter or sunflower seed butter
1 small firm banana (no brown spots), sliced
1½ teaspoons desiccated coconut, toasted
Drizzle of maple syrup

1 Toast the bread. Spread the nut or seed butter over the toast, top with sliced banana and toasted coconut. Add a drizzle of maple syrup to taste.

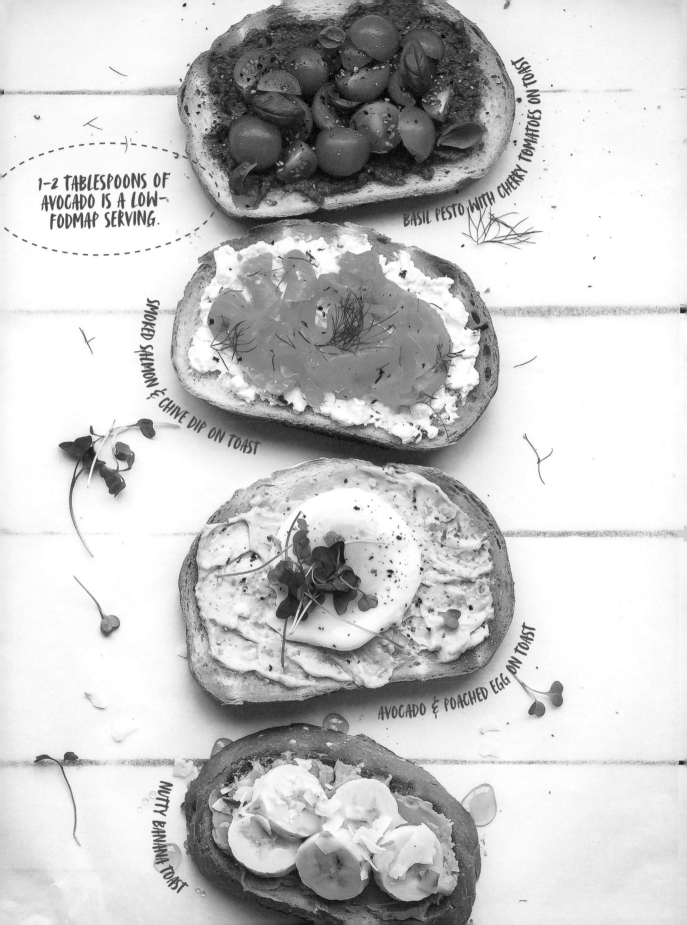

1-2 TABLESPOONS OF AVOCADO IS A LOW-FODMAP SERVING.

BASIL PESTO WITH CHERRY TOMATOES ON TOAST

SMOKED SALMON & CHIVE DIP ON TOAST

AVOCADO & POACHED EGG ON TOAST

NUTTY BANANA TOAST

Cinnamon French Toast

PREP TIME: 5 minutes COOK TIME: 20 minutes
SERVES: 4

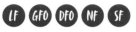

1 cup (250ml) low-FODMAP milk*

3 eggs

3 tablespoons brown sugar

2 teaspoons ground cinnamon

¼ teaspoon ground nutmeg

1 teaspoon vanilla essence

4 tablespoons dairy-free spread or
    butter, for cooking

8 slices low-FODMAP or gluten-free
    bread*

4 tablespoons pure maple syrup

4 servings of low-FODMAP fruit
    (e.g. strawberries, blueberries,
    raspberries, or firm banana)

Fluffy, sweet, and just a little bit crunchy . . . this low-FODMAP French toast recipe is sure to satisfy your sweet tooth!

1 In a large bowl, whisk together the milk, eggs, brown sugar, cinnamon, nutmeg, and vanilla essence.

2 Melt 1 tablespoon of the dairy-free spread or butter in a large frying pan over medium heat.

3 Dip each slice of bread in the batter until it is well covered but not too soggy, and place in the hot frying pan. Fry each side of the bread until golden brown. Cook the bread in batches (adding a little more spread or butter with each batch) and keep warm in the oven until ready to serve.

4 Top the warm French toast with maple syrup and a serving of low-FODMAP fruit. I love using strawberries if they are in season.

TIPS

It doesn't matter whether you use gluten-free bread or low-FODMAP sourdough bread, just make sure the bread isn't super fresh, otherwise your French toast might go soggy.

*Check buying tips (see pages 26–27).

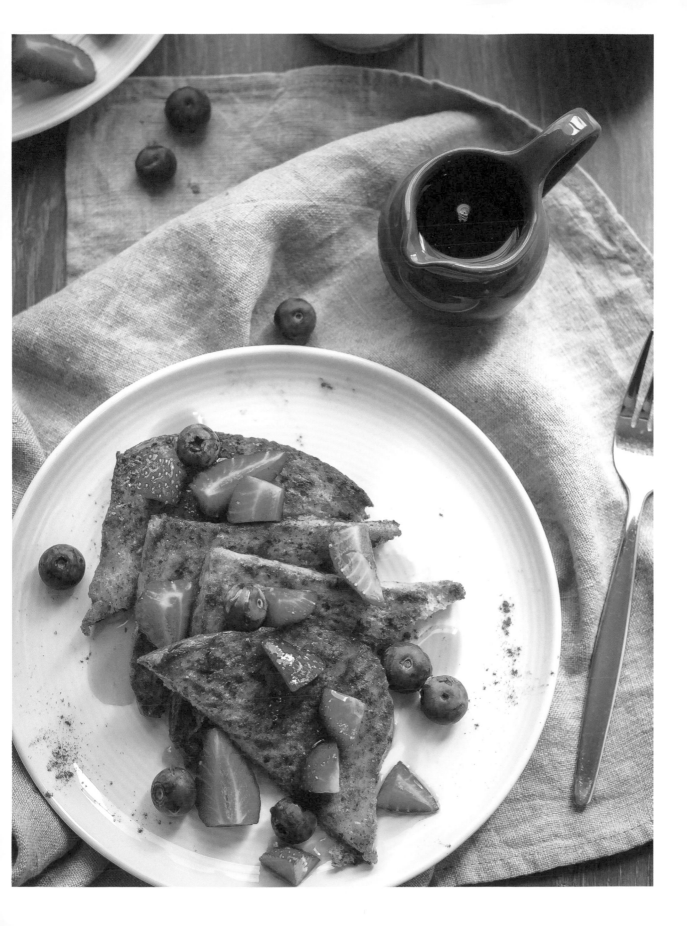

Caramelized Banana Oatmeal

COOK TIME: 7 minutes
SERVES: 1

(LF) (GFO) (DFO) (EF) (NFO) (SF)

½ cup rice flakes or rolled oats
½ cup (125ml) low-FODMAP milk*
   (double the milk if using oats)
2 teaspoons neutral oil (e.g. canola,
   grapeseed, safflower, sunflower)
2 teaspoons pure maple syrup
Sprinkle of ground cinnamon
¼ teaspoon vanilla essence
1 small firm banana (no brown spots),
   sliced

Warm up with a deliciously creamy oatmeal! Caramelized bananas bring a lovely sweetness to this dish, while the hints of cinnamon and vanilla remind me of my childhood breakfasts.

If you have celiac disease, choose rice flakes instead of rolled oats and boost your fiber intake by adding a tablespoon of low-FODMAP nuts or seeds or a teaspoon of chia seeds.

1 Cook the rice flakes or oats, according to package instructions, using low-FODMAP milk.

2 Heat a small saucepan over medium heat. Add the oil, maple syrup, cinnamon, and vanilla essence. Allow to bubble for 1 minute.

3 Add the sliced banana and cook for 2–3 minutes, until the banana is plump and golden.

4 Serve the caramelized banana on top of the oatmeal.

TIPS
*Check buying tips (see page 27).

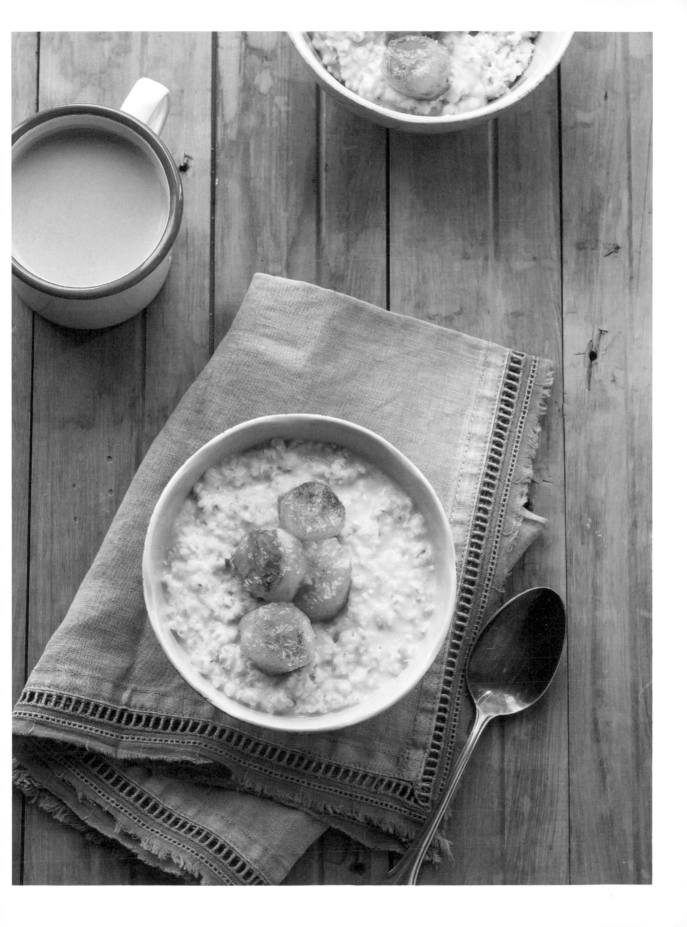

Curried Ground Beef on Toast

PREP TIME: 10 minutes COOK TIME: 20 minutes
SERVES: 4

LF GFO DF EF NF

2 tablespoons garlic-infused oil*

1 pound (450g) lean ground beef

3 teaspoons curry powder*

1 tablespoon soy sauce (GF if needed)

2 tablespoons tomato paste

1 cup (250ml) low-FODMAP chicken
  stock* (GF if needed)

1 teaspoon corn starch (GF if needed),
  dissolved in a small amount of cold
  water

4 cups (4oz/120g) baby spinach,
  chopped

2 large carrots (8½oz/240g), peeled
  and grated

¼ cup finely chopped scallions (green
  leaves only)

A few grinds of salt and pepper, to
  taste

8 slices low-FODMAP or gluten-free
  bread,* to serve

4 handfuls mixed lettuce leaves, to
  serve

The boys in my household love ground beef on toast for breakfast. It's filling, budget friendly, and full of flavor. This meal also makes a great light lunch or dinner option.

1 Heat a large nonstick frying pan over medium heat. Add the oil and ground beef. Cook until the beef has browned evenly.

2 Add the curry powder, soy sauce, and tomato paste to the beef and mix.

3 Turn the heat to medium–low. Stir in the chicken stock, corn starch, spinach, and carrot and mix. Allow the beef mixture to simmer and thicken. Stir in the scallion (reserve 1–2 tablespoons for garnish). Season well with salt and pepper.

4 Once the beef mixture has thickened, toast the bread. Top with a handful of mixed lettuce leaves and then a dollop of curried beef. Garnish with reserved scallions.

TIPS

This ground beef mixture will keep for 3 days in the fridge. Otherwise, pop the leftovers into the freezer and defrost in the microwave as needed.

*Check buying tips (see pages 25–26).

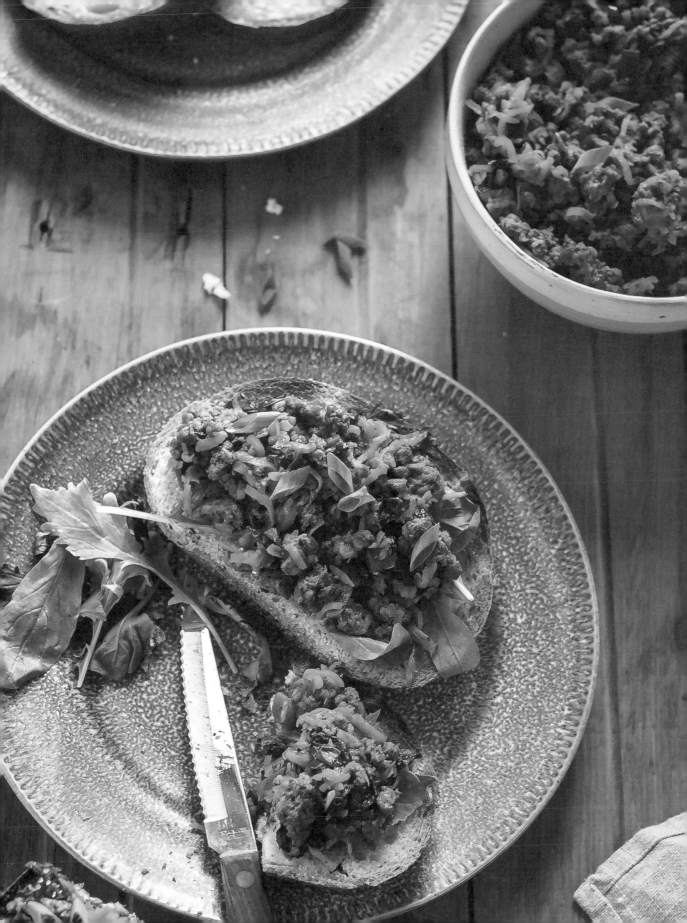

Mini Banana Pancakes

PREP TIME: 5 minutes **COOK TIME**: 20 minutes
MAKES: 8 small pancakes (serves 2–3)

LF GF DFO NF SF

2 small (5½oz/160g) firm bananas (no brown spots)
2 large eggs
¼ teaspoon baking powder (GF if needed)
A good pinch of salt
2 tablespoons gluten-free all-purpose flour*
½ teaspoon ground cinnamon
¼ teaspoon ground nutmeg
1 tablespoon brown sugar
3 tablespoons dairy-free spread or butter, for cooking
6 tablespoons coconut yogurt*
10 large blueberries
Sprinkle of confectioners' sugar (GF if needed, optional)

These pancakes make a deliciously filling breakfast. They aren't as light and fluffy as regular pancakes; instead, they are mini slices of banana bread in pancake form.

1 In a large bowl, mash the bananas until smooth, then whisk in the eggs. Add the baking powder, salt, flour, cinnamon, nutmeg, and brown sugar. Mix until well combined.

2 Heat a large frying pan over medium heat. Add a tablespoon of dairy-free spread or butter. Scoop 1–2 tablespoons of batter into the pan for each pancake. Allow the batter to cook until you see small bubbles forming on top. Peek underneath and if it's golden brown, gently flip it. Cook until both sides are golden brown.

3 Repeat until all the batter has been used. Add more dairy-free spread or butter to the pan as needed. If at any stage the pan becomes too hot, turn it down to medium–low.

4 Serve the pancakes with layers of coconut yogurt and blueberries. Dust with confectioners' sugar, if desired.

TIPS
*Check buying tips (see page 25).

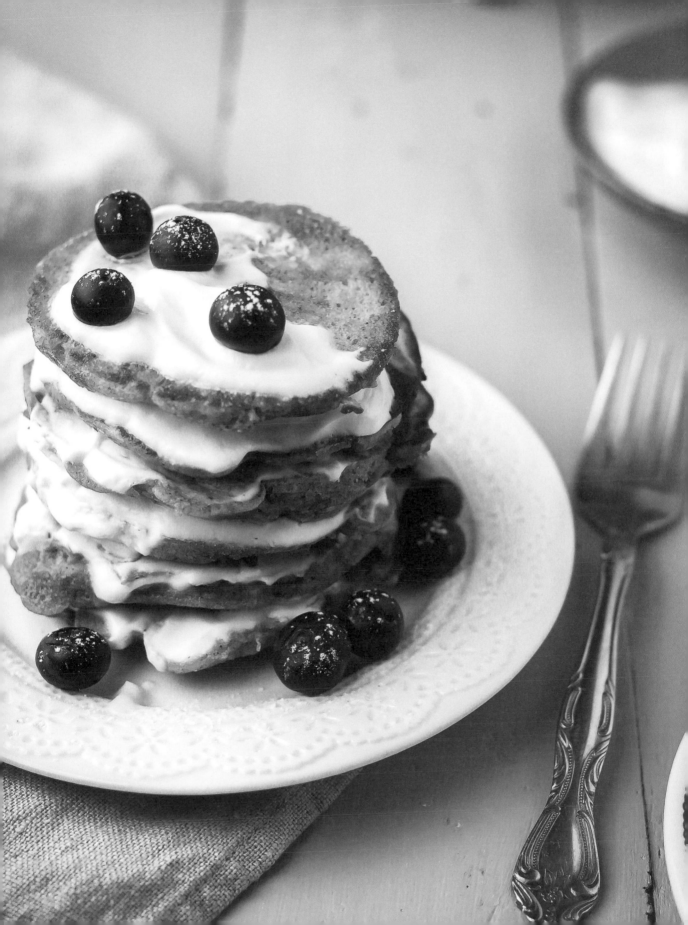

Magic Veggie Fritters

PREP TIME: 20 minutes COOK TIME: 25 minutes
MAKES: 12 (limit 3 fritters per serving)

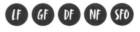

2 cups (12½oz/360g) grated potato

1 cup (8½oz/240g) grated zucchini

¾ cup (5½oz/160g) grated carrot

½ cup finely chopped scallions (green leaves only)

2 tablespoons finely chopped fresh parsley

½ teaspoon salt

1 tablespoon garlic-infused oil*

½ teaspoon paprika

¼ teaspoon ground turmeric

¼ teaspoon ground cumin

¼ cup (35g) gluten-free all-purpose flour*

¼ teaspoon black pepper

Zesty Lemon Aïoli (see recipe on page 212), to serve

Smoky Barbecue Sauce (see recipe on page 210), to serve

12 cherry tomatoes, lightly grilled, to serve

Handful of microgreens, to garnish

These fritters make tasty veggie-packed hash browns! They are perfect for breakfast or as a side for dinner.

1 Preheat oven to 400°F. Line a baking sheet with parchment paper.

2 Place half the potato, zucchini, and carrot in a clean tea towel and squeeze out all the excess liquid. Place in a clean bowl and repeat with remaining grated veggies (removing moisture helps create crispy fritters).

3 Place the grated veggies, scallions, parsley, salt, oil, paprika, turmeric, cumin, flour, and black pepper in a large bowl. Mix until well combined.

4 Using a ¼-cup measure, scoop up the mixture and shape into fritters. Place each one on the prepared baking sheet and flatten slightly.

5 Place the baking sheet in the middle of the oven. Bake for 15 minutes, then flip and cook for another 5–10 minutes, until golden brown and crunchy.

6 Serve hot with Zesty Lemon Aïoli or Smoky Barbecue Sauce and lightly grilled cherry tomatoes. Garnish with microgreens.

TIPS

These cook well on the barbecue. Just fry each fritter on the hotplate for a few minutes on each side until golden brown.

*Check buying tips (see page 25).

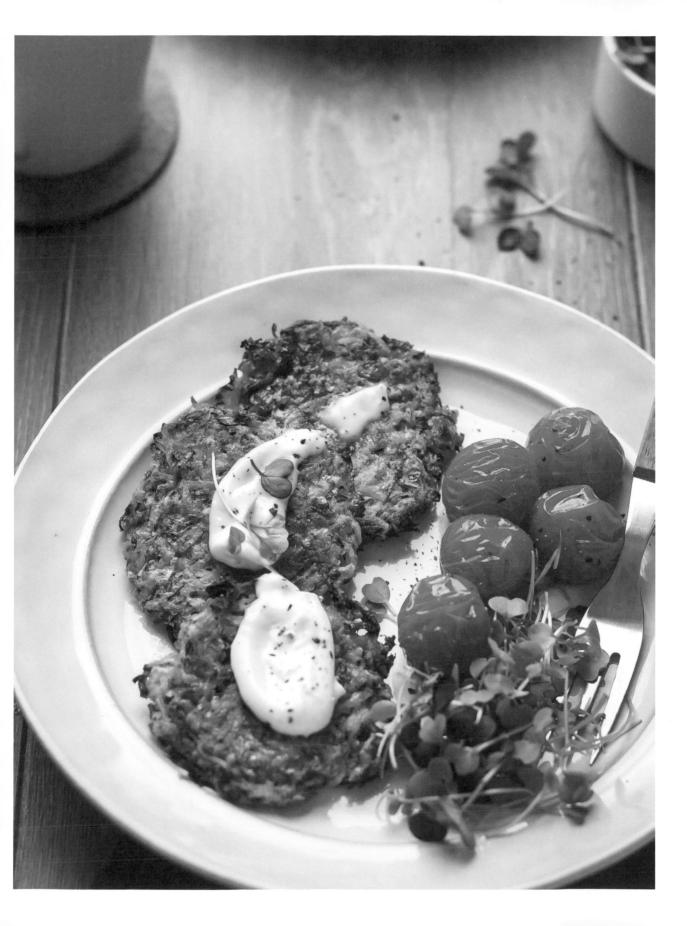

Chia Seed Bowls

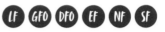

These are simple, delicious, and packed full of fiber. I suggest you start with one-third of a chia seed bowl and work your way up to a whole serving to allow your body to adjust to the fiber intake.

STRAWBERRY CHIA SEED BOWL

½ cup (2½oz/80g) fresh or frozen strawberries
1 ounce (30g) firm banana (no brown spots)
½ cup (125ml) low-FODMAP milk*
1 teaspoon lemon juice
½ teaspoon vanilla essence
1½ tablespoon chia seeds
1 teaspoon toasted pumpkin seeds, to serve
Sprinkle of toasted dried shredded coconut, to serve
Drizzle of maple syrup (optional)

1 Place the strawberries, banana, milk, lemon juice, and vanilla essence in a blender and blend together until smooth. Mix in the chia seeds. Place in the fridge to set overnight or for at least 6 hours (it should be like slightly runny jam). Serve with pumpkin seeds and coconut. Add a dash of maple syrup, if desired.

VANILLA PASSIONFRUIT CHIA SEED BOWL

1½ tablespoons chia seeds
½ cup (125ml) low-FODMAP milk*
1 teaspoon pure maple syrup
½ teaspoon vanilla essence
1 passionfruit, to serve
1 tablespoon toasted dried shredded coconut, to serve

1 Mix the chia seeds, milk, maple syrup, and vanilla essence together and place in the fridge to set overnight. Serve with passionfruit pulp and coconut. Add another dash of maple syrup or vanilla to taste, if desired.

CHOCOLATE CHIA SEED BREAKFAST BOWL

½ cup (125ml) low-FODMAP milk*
¾ tablespoon unsweetened cocoa powder (GF if needed)
½ teaspoon pure maple syrup or ¼ teaspoon stevia powder
½ teaspoon vanilla essence
2 tablespoons chia seeds
1 serving of low-FODMAP fruit (e.g. sliced firm banana, strawberries, raspberries, blueberries)

1 Whisk the milk, cocoa powder, maple syrup or stevia, and vanilla essence together until smooth. Mix in the chia seeds. Place in the fridge to set overnight. Serve with low-FODMAP fruit and add extra maple syrup to taste.

TIPS
*Check buying tips (see page 27).

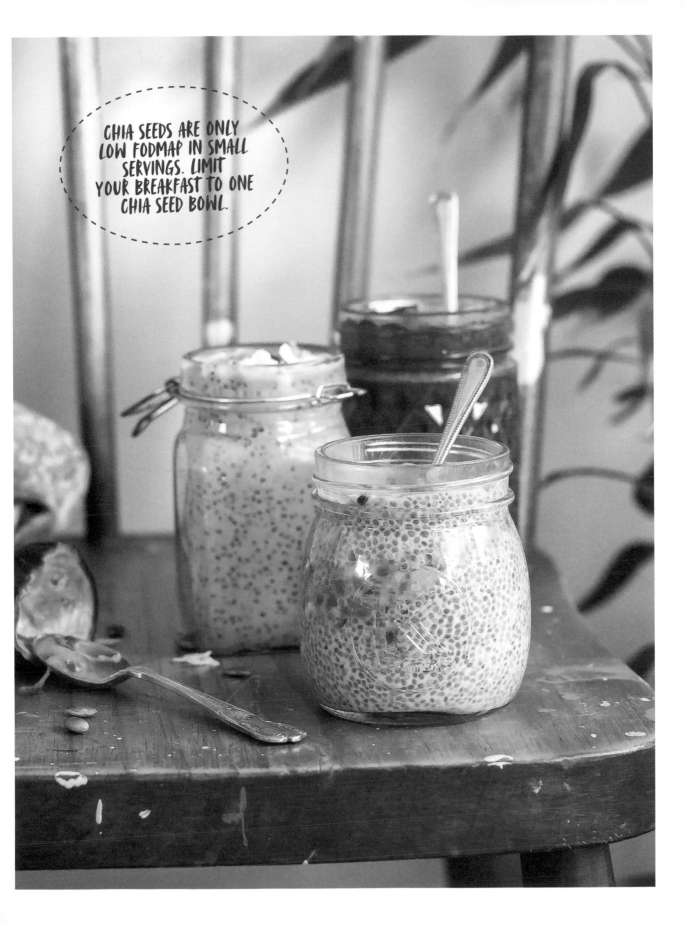

CHIA SEEDS ARE ONLY
LOW FODMAP IN SMALL
SERVINGS. LIMIT
YOUR BREAKFAST TO ONE
CHIA SEED BOWL.

Saucy Egg Shakshuka

PREP TIME: 15 minutes **COOK TIME**: 20 minutes
SERVES: 4

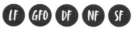

1 tablespoon garlic-infused oil*

1 red bell pepper, seeded and cut into strips

1 (15oz/400g) can plain crushed/chopped tomatoes

1 cup (250ml) low-FODMAP chicken stock* (GF if needed)

1 tablespoon corn starch (GF if needed)

2 cups (2oz/60g) baby spinach, roughly chopped

¼ cup finely chopped scallions (green leaves only)

1 teaspoon paprika

1 teaspoon ground cumin

⅛ teaspoon crushed red pepper*

½ teaspoon white sugar

A few grinds of salt and pepper, to taste

4 large eggs

2 tablespoons chopped, fresh flat-leaf parsley

8 slices low-FODMAP or gluten-free bread,* to serve

This egg dish makes the perfect weekend breakfast. It has plenty of flavor without being too spicy. My favorite part is dipping toast into the shakshuka sauce.

As always, remember to divide the recipe into the recommended number of servings.

1 Heat the oil in a large frying pan over medium–high heat. Add the bell pepper and fry until it starts to soften.

2 Pour in the tomatoes and chicken stock. Mix and simmer the sauce for 2 minutes. Dissolve the corn starch in a small amount of warm water and mix into the sauce, along with the spinach and the scallions.

3 Cook for another 2 minutes, until the sauce starts to thicken. Add the paprika, cumin, crushed red pepper, and sugar. Season with salt and pepper. Taste and add more of the spices if desired, then turn down the heat to medium–low.

4 Crack the eggs into the tomato mixture, spacing them evenly around the frying pan. Cover and simmer for 10–15 minutes, until the eggs are cooked to your liking.

5 Sprinkle with fresh parsley and serve with a side of toasted low-FODMAP bread.

TIPS
*Check buying tips (see pages 25–26).

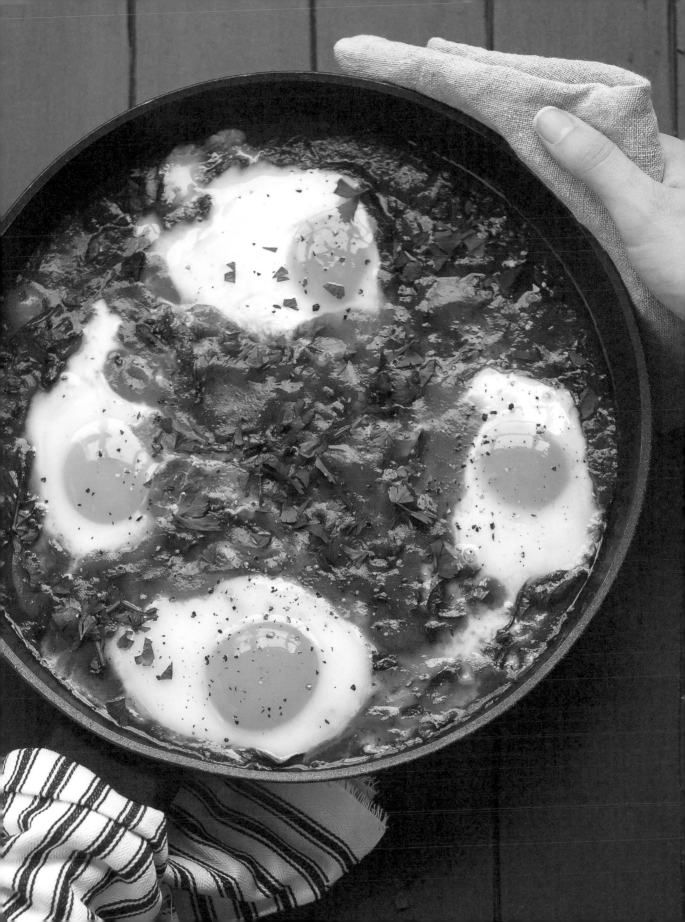

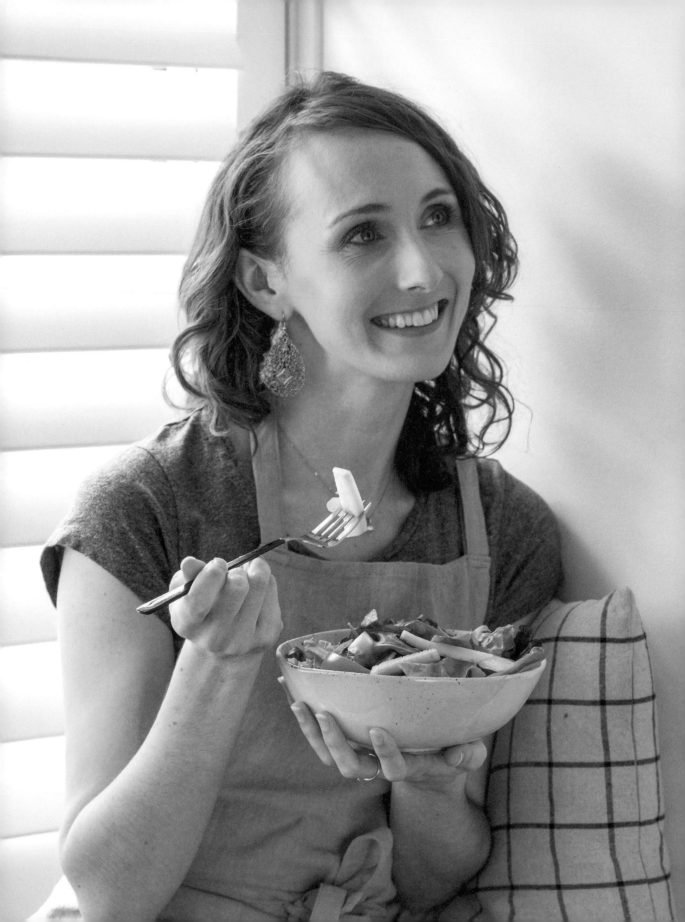

LUNCH

Whether you like a classic sandwich, a fresh salad, homemade soup, or a tasty fritter, I've got you covered.

Crunchy Thai Brown Rice Salad

PREP TIME: 10 minutes COOK TIME: 30 minutes
SERVES: 4

LF GFO DF EF NFO

1¼ cups long-grain brown rice

THAI SALAD

1½ cups (8oz/225g) frozen edamame
   beans
4 tablespoons sunflower and pumpkin
   seeds, to garnish
2 cups (6oz/180g) finely shredded red
   cabbage
1 cup (2½oz/75g) finely shredded
   iceberg lettuce
1 large (4oz/120g) carrot, peeled and
   grated
½ cup fresh flat-leaf parsley
¼ cup finely sliced scallions (green
   leaves only)

MOCK PEANUT DRESSING

¼ cup sunflower seed butter or
   peanut butter
2½ tablespoons soy sauce (GF if
   needed)
1 tablespoon pure maple syrup
1 tablespoon rice wine vinegar
1 teaspoon sesame seeds
½ teaspoon crushed ginger*
1 tablespoon lemon juice
¼ teaspoon crushed red pepper*
A few grinds of salt and pepper, to
   taste

This crunchy salad is perfect for lunch or for nights when
you just want an easy vegan meal. I made this recipe nut-
free by creating a mock peanut sauce using sunflower seed
butter (you might need to shop around until you find one you
enjoy), but you can use regular peanut butter if you wish. You
can enjoy this salad warm or cold, and the leftovers make a
fantastic packed lunch.

1 Cook the brown rice according to package instructions.

2 Place the edamame beans in a bowl of warm water to thaw.
Drain after a few minutes.

3 Toast the sunflower and pumpkin seeds in a small saucepan
over medium heat until golden brown.

4 To make the dressing, melt the sunflower seed butter or
peanut butter in the microwave for 20 seconds, then whisk in
the soy sauce, maple syrup, vinegar, sesame seeds, ginger,
lemon juice, and crushed red pepper. Taste and season with
salt and pepper as desired. If the dressing is too thick, whisk in
a little water.

5 Place the cooked brown rice, salad vegetables, and
dressing in a large bowl. Toss well to combine, then top with
toasted sunflower and pumpkin seeds.

TIPS
*Check buying tips (see page 25).

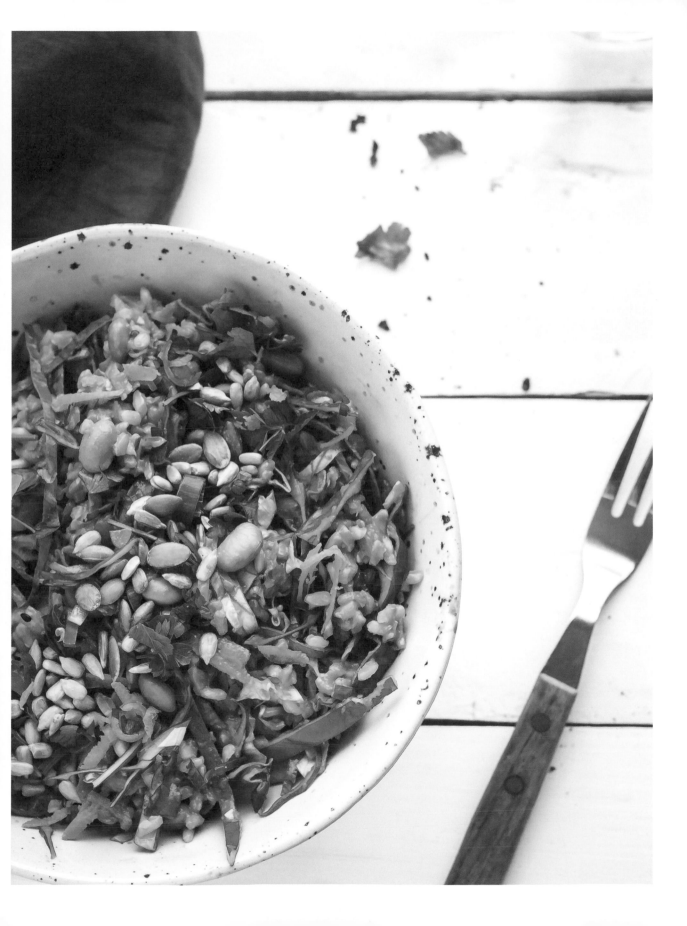

Summer Beef Salad with Mustard Vinaigrette

PREP TIME: 15 minutes COOK TIME: 15 minutes
SERVES: 4

LF · GF · DF · EF · NF · SF

1 red bell pepper, halved and seeded

1¼ pounds (550g) beef rump steak or sirloin steak

1 tablespoon neutral oil (e.g. canola, grapeseed, safflower, sunflower)

A few grinds of salt and pepper

1½ cups (6oz/180g) chopped green beans

6 cups shredded lettuce (e.g. butter, iceberg, red leaf)

16 cherry tomatoes, halved

¼ cup finely sliced scallions (green leaves only)

MUSTARD VINAIGRETTE

1½ tablespoons Dijon mustard*

2 tablespoons white vinegar

¼ cup (60ml) olive oil

¼ teaspoon black pepper

¼ teaspoon white sugar

You can't beat a yummy salad on a hot day. Thinly sliced beef with cherry tomatoes and a mustard vinaigrette makes for a delicious combo.

1 Grill the bell pepper in the oven until the skin starts to blacken. Leave to cool. Loosen the skin with your fingers, then slide a blunt knife under the skin and peel it off. Discard the blackened skin and cut the red flesh into strips.

2 Season the steak by rubbing each side with oil, salt, and pepper. Heat a large frying pan over medium–high heat and cook the steak for 4 minutes on each side for medium-rare, or until cooked to your liking. Allow to rest for 5 minutes before thinly slicing.

3 While the steak cooks, blanch the green beans in boiling water for 2 minutes (they should turn bright green and tender). Drain and rinse under cold water, then drain again.

4 To make the vinaigrette, mix all the dressing ingredients together in a small bowl or jar until smooth. If too sour, try adding a couple of pinches of sugar until it is sweet enough.

5 Assemble the salad ingredients and serve the sliced steak on top. Drizzle with the vinaigrette.

TIPS
*Check buying tips (see page 26).

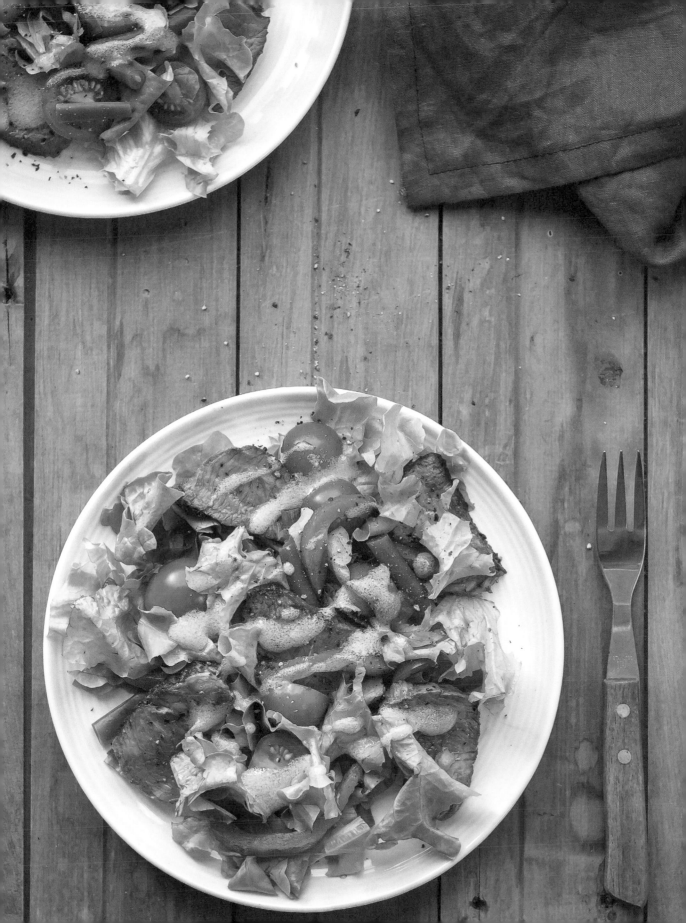

Simple Potato & Egg Salad

PREP TIME: 10 minutes **COOK TIME:** 25 minutes
SERVES: 4

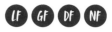

1¾ pounds (800g) potatoes, peeled and diced

1¼ cups (5½oz/160g) chopped green beans

4 large eggs

1 red bell pepper, seeded and diced

1 small cucumber, peeled and cut into sticks

3 tablespoons finely chopped scallions (green leaves only)

3 tablespoons finely chopped fresh chives

DRESSING

1 tablespoon wholegrain mustard*

⅓ cup (85ml) mayonnaise

1 tablespoon lemon juice

A few grinds of black pepper

This simple salad makes a nutritious and delicious lunch or side dish for a family barbecue. It tastes so good, no one will ever know it is low FODMAP!

1 Boil the potatoes in water until tender. Add the green beans to the saucepan about 3 minutes before you drain the potatoes. Cook the green beans for 2–3 minutes, until tender and brightly colored. Drain and set aside to cool.

2 While the potatoes cook, hard-boil the eggs. Place the eggs in a small saucepan of water and cover with cold water. Bring the water to a rolling boil over medium–high heat. Boil for 2 minutes before turning the heat down to the lowest setting. Cook for 10–12 minutes. Drain the eggs and run under cold water before peeling. Cut into quarters.

3 To make the dressing, mix together the mustard, mayonnaise, lemon juice, and black pepper in a small bowl or jar.

4 In a large bowl, gently mix together the potatoes, green beans, hard-boiled eggs, bell pepper, cucumber, scallions, chives, and salad dressing. Season with a few grinds of black pepper.

TIPS
*Check buying tips (see page 26).

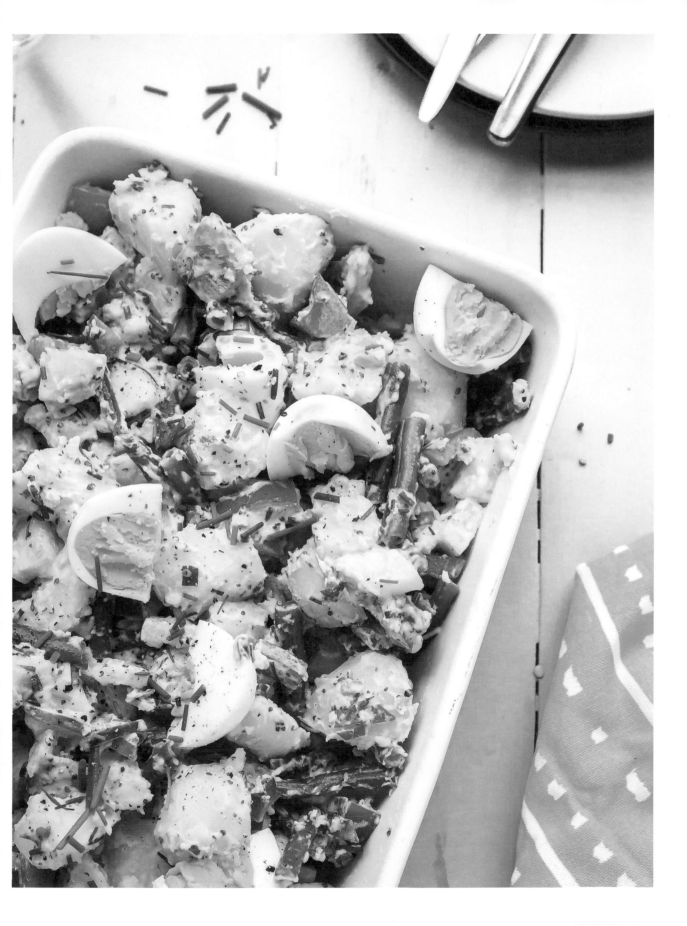

Roasted Veggie & Brown Rice Salad

PREP TIME: 10 minutes **COOK TIME:** 30 minutes
SERVES: 4

LF GF DFO EF NF SF

1 cup medium-grain brown rice (or
   2 cups cooked brown rice)

2 cups (2½oz/75g) arugula

3 cups sliced leftover Gorgeous Roasted
   Veggies (see recipe on page 198)

3 tablespoons finely chopped parsley

½ cup finely chopped scallions (green
   leaves only)

3 tablespoons crumbled feta (optional)

3 tablespoons toasted pumpkin seeds
   or pine nuts (optional)

A few grinds of salt and pepper, to
   taste

DRESSING

1½ tablespoons balsamic vinegar

1½ tablespoons lemon juice

3 tablespoons extra virgin olive oil

Pinch of white sugar

Brown rice salads make awesome take-to-work options and
are a fantastic way to use up leftover veggies.

1 Cook the brown rice according to package instructions.

2 Place the arugula, roasted veggies, parsley, and scallions
in a large bowl and toss in the cooked rice. Add the feta and
pumpkin seeds or pine nuts, if using.

3 To make the dressing, mix all the dressing ingredients
together in a small bowl or jar. Pour over the salad and gently
mix. Season with salt and pepper.

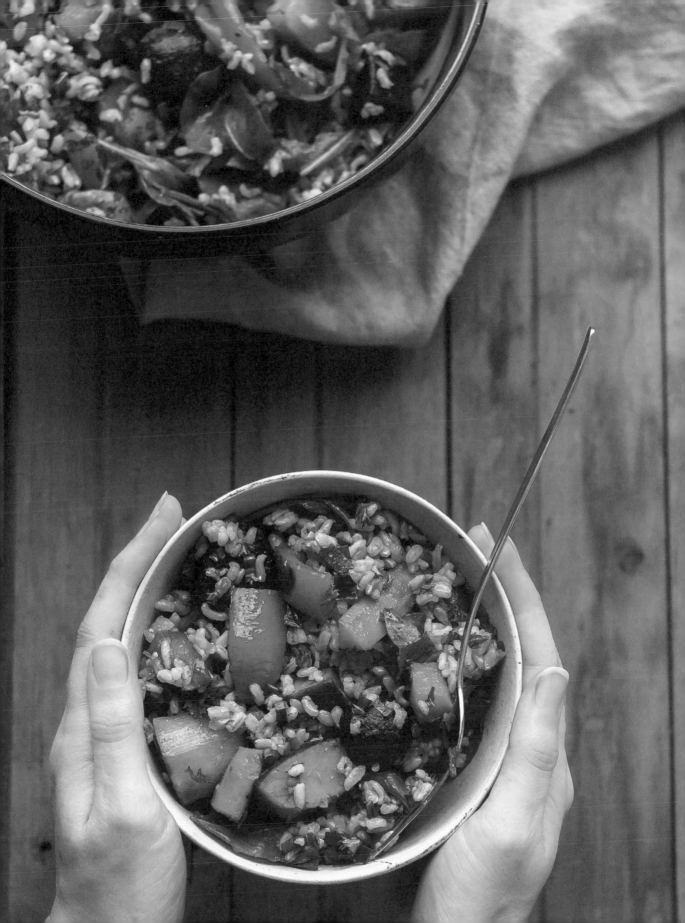

Moroccan Chicken Mason Jar Salad

PREP TIME: 5 minutes COOK TIME: 10 minutes
SERVES: 2

LF GF DF EF NF SF

MOROCCAN CHICKEN

½ pound (250g) skinless chicken
    breast
½ tablespoon garlic-infused oil*
1½ teaspoons Moroccan Spice Mix
    (see recipe on page 211)
A few grinds of salt and pepper

ORANGE DRESSING

2 tablespoons olive oil
1 tablespoon freshly squeezed orange
    juice
½ tablespoon pure maple syrup
½ tablespoon red wine vinegar
¼ teaspoon salt
A few grinds of black pepper

SALAD

1 red bell pepper, seeded and diced
1 small cucumber, peeled, cut in half
    lengthwise, and sliced
2 mandarins, peeled and separated
2 cups shredded assorted lettuce
    leaves

This Moroccan-inspired salad is quick and easy to throw together. Each serving fits perfectly into a 1-pint Mason jar, which makes it super convenient to take to work!

1 Cut the chicken into cubes and place in a bowl. Add the oil and spice mix. Combine until the chicken is well coated. Season with salt and pepper.

2 Heat a nonstick frying pan over medium–high heat. Stir-fry the chicken for 3–4 minutes, until golden brown and cooked through. Set aside to cool. If possible, cook the chicken the night before and leave to cool in the fridge.

3 To make the dressing, mix together all the ingredients in a small bowl or jar.

4 Prepare the salad ingredients.

5 If using Mason jars, assemble the salad in the jars in this order: orange dressing, bell pepper, cucumber, chicken, mandarin, and lettuce.

6 To serve, gently shake the jar (with the lid on) to coat the salad in dressing and eat straight from the jar. Alternatively, tip the salad onto a plate.

TIPS
*Check buying tips (see page 25).

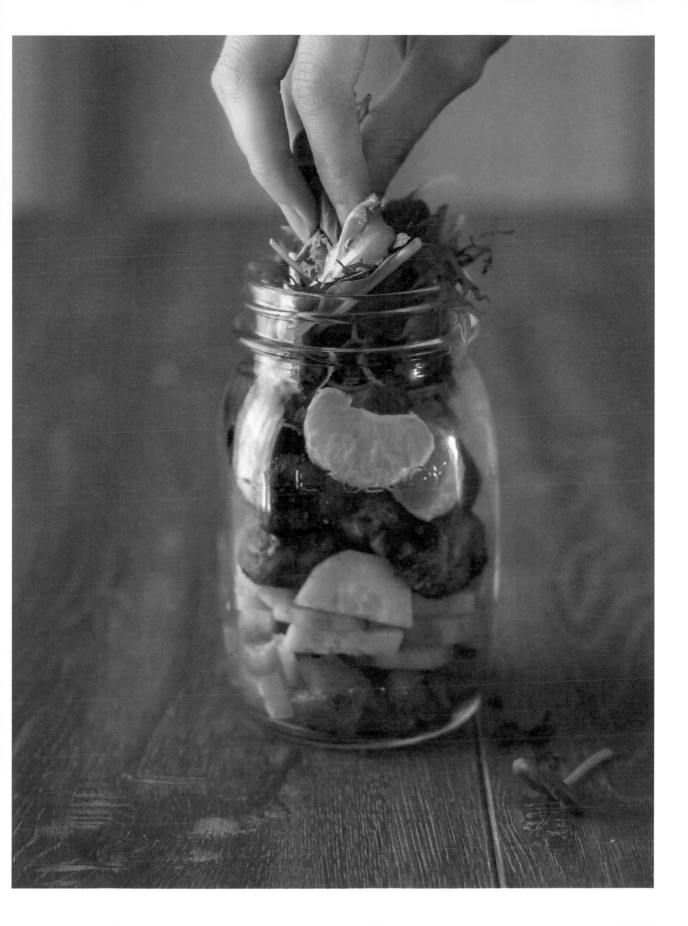

Classic Green Salad with Italian Dressing

PREP TIME: 15 minutes
SERVES: 6

LF GF DF EF NF SF

5–6 cups assorted lettuce leaves

3 medium tomatoes, cut into wedges

1 small cucumber, peeled and cut into chunky sticks

2 radishes, thinly sliced

1 red bell pepper, seeded and diced

2 cups cooked protein (e.g. chicken, beef, tofu) (optional)

ITALIAN DRESSING

Makes 1 cup; use 1–2 tablespoons per serving

¾ cup extra virgin olive oil

3½ tablespoons red wine vinegar

2 teaspoons garlic-infused oil*

½ teaspoon black pepper

½ teaspoon salt

¾ teaspoon dried oregano

½ teaspoon dried basil

¼ teaspoon crushed red pepper*

1 teaspoon sugar

TIPS

Store the Italian dressing in the fridge for up to 3 weeks. If the olive oil turns solid in the fridge, bring the dressing up to room temperature for 30 minutes and then stir well before using.

*Check buying tips (see page 25).

Simple food is good food and you can't go wrong with a classic green salad. Most store-bought Italian dressings contain high-FODMAP ingredients, so in this recipe I teach you how to make your own.

1 Toss together the salad ingredients. Place in individual containers for grab-and-go lunches or on a platter for a side dish.

2 To make the dressing, whisk all the ingredients together in a glass jar and leave to infuse for at least 30 minutes before using. Taste and add another splash of red wine vinegar, if desired.

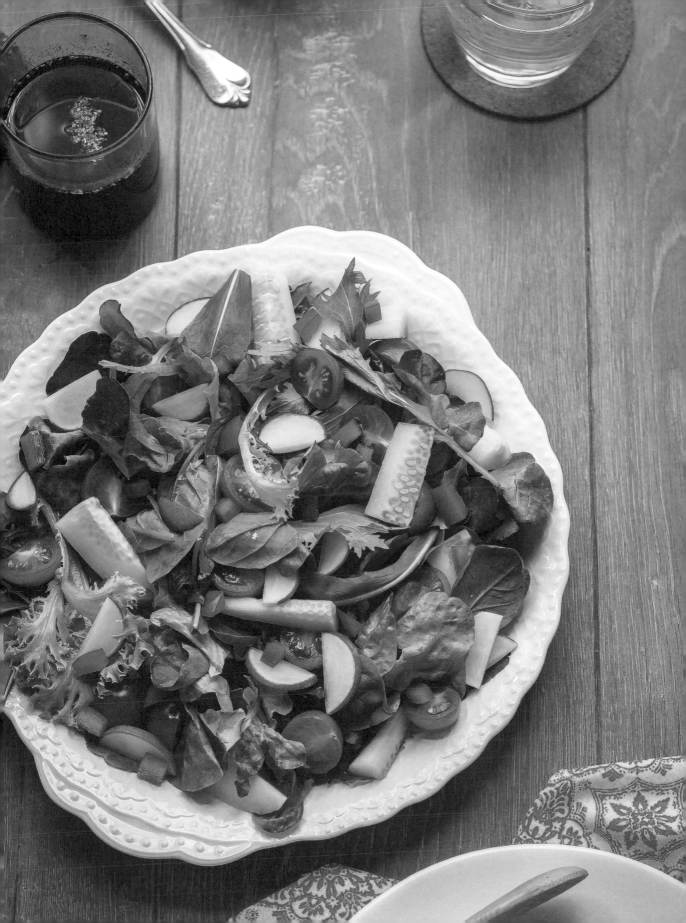

Caramelized Beet, Pumpkin & Feta Salad

PREP TIME: 10 minutes **COOK TIME**: 35 minutes
SERVES: 4

LF GF DFO EF NF SF

10½ ounces (300g) kabocha squash/
  Japanese pumpkin, peeled and
  seeded
Drizzle of olive oil
A few grinds of salt and pepper
8 ounces (240g) canned whole beets,
  drained and patted dry (weigh after
  draining)
¼ cup mixed sunflower and sesame
  seeds
½ teaspoon paprika
1 teaspoon olive oil
3 cups mixed lettuce leaves
Large handful of baby mint leaves
2–3 tablespoons feta, crumbled
  (optional)

CARAMELIZED SAUCE

1 tablespoon dairy-free spread or
  butter
2 tablespoons brown sugar
¼ cup (60ml) freshly squeezed orange
  juice (1 large orange)
2 teaspoons orange zest
⅛ teaspoon ground cinnamon

This salad has beautiful bursts of orange flavor and hints of cinnamon, which I adore. Don't skimp on the mint leaves, as these really help to draw out the flavor. I love having this salad as a light lunch or using it as a side for dinner parties.

1 Preheat oven to 400°F. Cut the pumpkin into ¾-inch pieces. Place in a roasting pan and toss with olive oil. Season with salt and pepper. Add the beets. Roast in the oven for 20–25 minutes, until the pumpkin is golden brown, turning once during cooking.

2 In a small bowl, mix together the sunflower and sesame seeds, paprika, and olive oil. Fry in a dry pan over medium heat until golden. Tip out onto a plate and set aside.

3 Once the pumpkin is cooked, remove from the oven, cool, and cut the beets into quarters.

4 To make the caramelized sauce, melt the dairy-free spread or butter in a large frying pan over medium heat. Whisk in the brown sugar, orange juice and zest, and cinnamon.

5 Once the sauce starts to thicken, add the roasted beets and pumpkin. Cook for 2–3 minutes, until the roasted veggies are coated and most of the caramelized sauce has been absorbed.

6 Toss the caramelized pumpkin and beets with the lettuce leaves, then garnish with the mint leaves, crispy seeds, and crumbled feta, if desired.

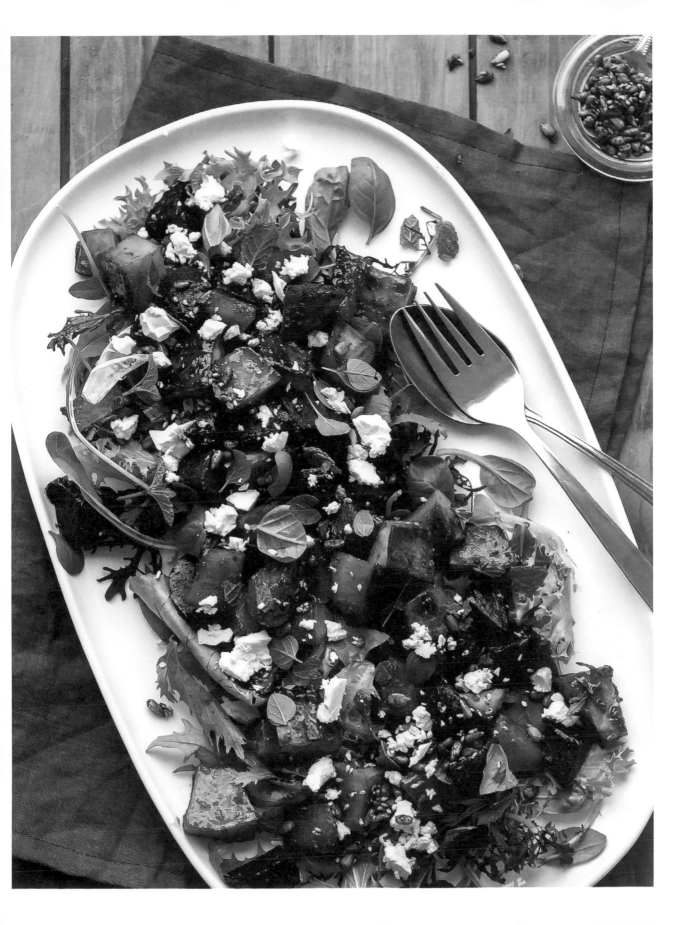

Cheesy Scones

PREP TIME: 15 minutes COOK TIME: 25 minutes
MAKES: 12 scones (limit 2 per serving)

LF GF DFO EF NF SFO

2 cups (280g) gluten-free self-rising
    flour*
½ cup (2oz/55g) grated Cheddar or
    vegan cheese*
¾ cup finely chopped scallions (green
    leaves only)
3 teaspoons baking powder (GF if
    needed)
½ teaspoon dried oregano
½ teaspoon dried rosemary
1 teaspoon salt
½ cup (125ml) low-FODMAP milk*
Drizzle of olive oil
Dairy-free spread or butter, to serve

These yummy savory scones are full of cheesy goodness and make a hearty lunch. The smell of them cooking is sure to bring the family rushing to the table. I recommend serving them hot, with plenty of butter and a bowl of Sweet Red Pepper Soup (see page 86).

1 Preheat oven to 350°F. Line a baking sheet with parchment paper.

2 In a large bowl, mix together all the ingredients except the milk and olive oil.

3 Slowly add the milk, mixing as you go, until the scone dough holds together. If the mixture is too dry, add another 1–2 tablespoons of milk. Sprinkle some flour on the countertop and knead the dough until it becomes relatively smooth. If the dough is too sticky, add another sprinkle of flour and work it in.

4 Place the scone dough on the prepared baking sheet. Shape it into a large oval about ½ inch thick. Then cut into 12 scones and gently separate, so they have room to rise.

5 Brush the top of each scone with olive oil and place in the middle of the oven. Cook for 20–25 minutes, until golden brown and a toothpick inserted into the middle comes out clean.

6 Serve hot with a generous amount of dairy-free spread or butter.

TIPS
These scones are best served hot, so reheat them in the microwave for 20–30 seconds before serving, or cut in half and grill in the oven.

*Check buying tips (see pages 25–27).

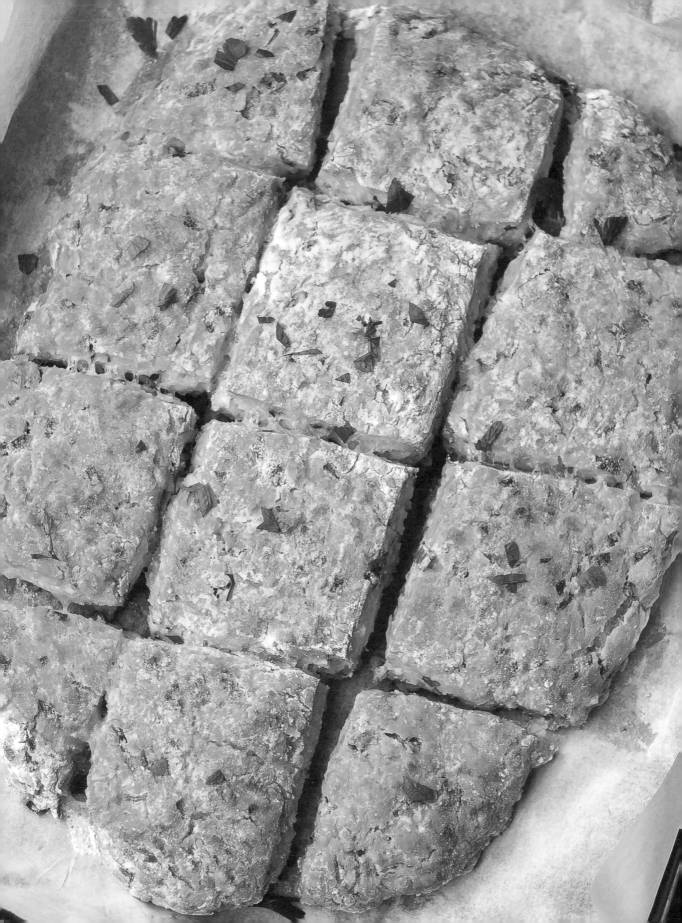

Cheesy Chicken Fritters

LF **GF** **DFO** **NF** **SFO**

1¼ pound (550g) ground chicken

2 large eggs

¼ cup (60ml) mayonnaise

¼ cup (35g) gluten-free all-purpose
   flour*

¾ cup (3oz/85g) grated mozzarella or
   vegan cheese*

2 tablespoons finely chopped fresh
   basil

2 teaspoons dried chives

¼ teaspoon salt

A few grinds of black pepper

Drizzle of olive oil, for cooking

Zesty Lemon Aïoli (see recipe on page
   212), to serve

When you are craving take-out chicken, try these fritters instead! They are insanely easy to make and super tasty. Just make sure you have some friends around to share them with, otherwise you might end up eating the whole batch by yourself . . .

1 Place the chicken, eggs, mayonnaise, flour, cheese, basil, chives, salt, and pepper in a bowl. Stir until well combined.

2 Heat a large nonstick frying pan over medium heat and add a drizzle of olive oil (about 1 tablespoon). Once the oil is hot, measure out ¼-cup scoops of the mixture and place in the pan. Flatten the mixture slightly with a spatula.

3 Fry each side for 3–4 minutes, until golden brown. Add more oil as needed. Once the chicken is fully cooked, place the fritters on a plate lined with a paper towel to drain. Cook the fritters in two or three batches.

4 Serve the fritters hot with a side of Zesty Lemon Aïoli.

TIPS
*Check buying tips (see page 25–26).

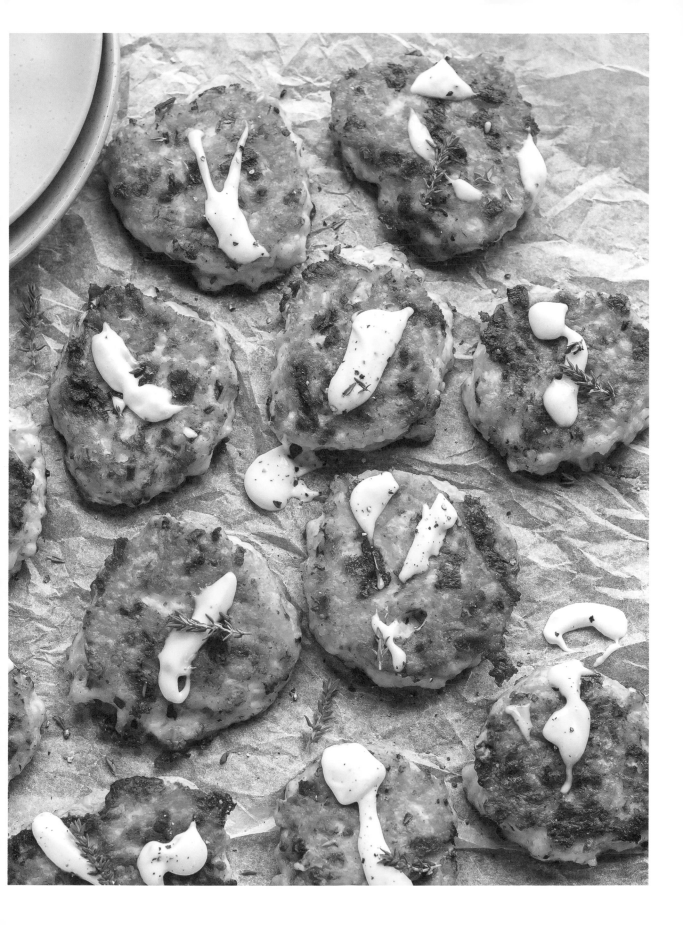

Curry Quinoa Fritters

PREP TIME: 20 minutes COOK TIME: 20 minutes
MAKES: 8 fritters (serves 2–3)

LF GF DF NF SFO

⅓ cup white quinoa

½ tablespoon olive oil

¾ cup (185ml) low-FODMAP chicken or vegetable stock* (GF if needed)

3 large eggs

¼ cup (35g) gluten-free all-purpose flour*

¼ teaspoon mild curry powder*

½ teaspoon paprika

1 medium/large (3oz/100g) carrot, peeled and grated

1 tablespoon finely chopped fresh chives

1 tablespoon finely chopped fresh cilantro

¼ cup finely chopped scallions (green leaves only)

A few grinds of salt and pepper

Zesty Lemon Aïoli (see recipe on page 212), to serve

Chopped fresh chives, to serve

These fritters make a tasty take-to-work lunch or party appetizer. The hint of curry and the fresh herbs go perfectly with the carrot and quinoa in the fritters.

1 Place the quinoa in a fine-meshed sieve and rinse under running water for 40 seconds (this will help remove the bitter taste). Place the quinoa in a medium saucepan with the olive oil and toast for 1 minute over medium–high heat.

2 Add the chicken or vegetable stock and bring to a rolling boil. Turn down the heat to medium–low and simmer until cooked (about 12–15 minutes). Remove from heat once the quinoa is soft (it's okay if it's still a little wet).

3 Whisk the eggs and flour in a large bowl until mostly smooth (a few flour lumps are okay). Add the curry powder, paprika, carrot, chives, cilantro, and scallions. Mix well, then stir in the cooked quinoa. Season generously with salt and pepper.

4 Heat a large frying pan over medium heat. When the frying pan is hot, measure out ¼-cup scoops of the mixture and place in the pan. Fry for 3–4 minutes on each side, until golden. Cook the fritters in two batches.

5 Serve with Zesty Lemon Aïoli and some extra chopped fresh chives.

TIPS
*Check buying tips (see pages 25–26).

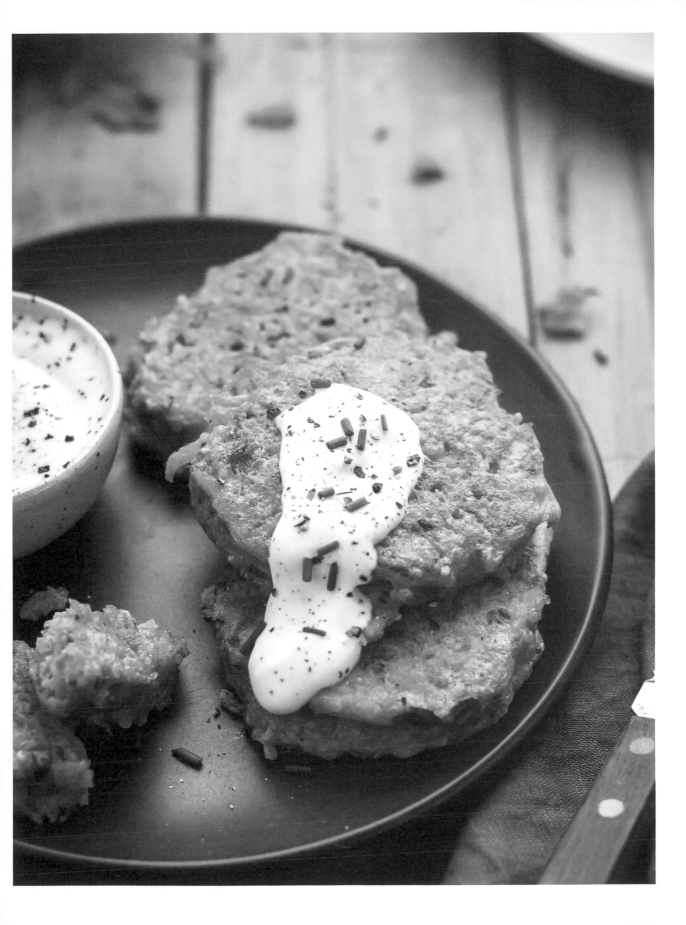

Crunchy Falafel

PREP TIME: 15 minutes **COOK TIME**: 25 minutes
SERVES: 5

(LF) (GF) (DF) (NF) (SFO)

2 medium (4oz/120g) carrots, peeled and grated

1 cup (6oz/170g) canned chickpeas (measure after draining and rinsing)

Zest and juice of 1 large lime

1 cup finely chopped fresh parsley

1 cup (2½oz/80g) finely chopped leeks (green leaves only)

1 cup microwave medium-grain brown rice or cooked brown rice

1 tablespoon garlic-infused oil*

1 teaspoon paprika

¾ teaspoon ground cumin

A few grinds of salt and pepper

4 tablespoons gluten-free all-purpose flour*

2 tablespoons olive oil, for cooking

Zesty Lemon Aïoli or Maple Mustard Dressing (see pages 212 and 213), to serve

These golden falafel medallions are a great vegetarian option while on the low-FODMAP diet. They're tasty, soft, and crunchy! I love serving these with a side salad or as a burger patty on a low-FODMAP bun. They are cooked in the oven, which is such an easy method when you are feeling lazy and want crispy falafel.

1 Preheat oven to 375°F. Line a baking sheet with parchment paper.

2 Place all the ingredients except the flour and cooking oil in a food processor. Blend until a smooth paste has formed (if the mixture is too dry, add a tablespoon of water). Once well combined, stir in the flour (the paste should become just dry enough to handle).

3 Grease the parchment paper with 1 tablespoon of olive oil (this helps the falafel go crispy). Scoop out the falafel using a tablespoon measure and form into small patties. Space them evenly on the baking sheet. Brush the tops with the other tablespoon of oil.

4 Bake for about 12 minutes on each side, until golden brown.

5 Serve with a side salad and Maple Mustard Dressing or Zesty Lemon Aïoli.

TIPS
*Check buying tips (see page 25).

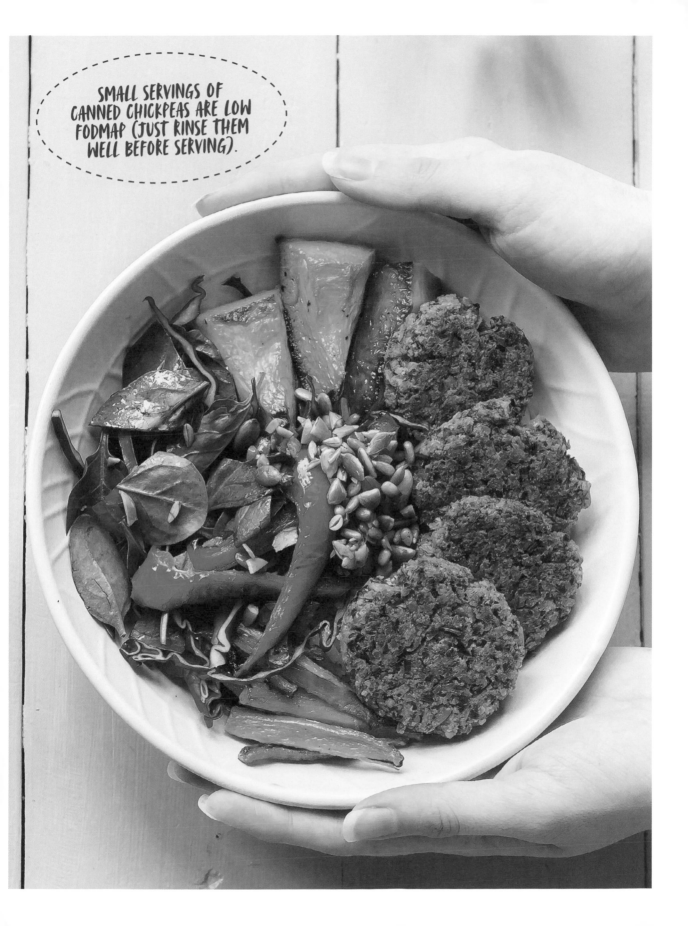

SMALL SERVINGS OF CANNED CHICKPEAS ARE LOW FODMAP (JUST RINSE THEM WELL BEFORE SERVING).

Mini Frittata Muffins

PREP TIME: 20 minutes **COOK TIME**: 20 minutes
MAKES: 12 mini frittatas (limit 3 per serving)

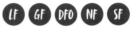

Drizzle of neutral oil (e.g. canola, grapeseed, safflower, sunflower)

5 ounces (150g) bacon, diced*

½ cup (1oz/40g) finely diced leeks (green leaves only)

9 eggs

¼ cup (60ml) low-FODMAP milk*

3 tablespoons gluten-free all-purpose flour*

¼ cup finely chopped fresh chives

Pinch of crushed red pepper*

2 cups (2oz/60g) finely chopped spinach

2 medium (4oz/120g) carrots, peeled and grated

A few grinds of salt and pepper

16 cherry tomatoes, halved

These mini frittatas are tasty and filling. The combination of chives and green leek tips gives them an oniony taste while keeping them low FODMAP.

1 Preheat oven to 375°F. Grease a 12-hole standard muffin pan.

2 Heat oil in a large frying pan over medium–high heat. Add the bacon and leeks and cook for 6–8 minutes (until the bacon starts to crisp).

3 Crack the eggs into a large bowl and whisk in the milk. Whisk in the flour (don't worry if the mixture stays a little lumpy). Stir in the chives, crushed red pepper, spinach, and carrot. Season with salt and pepper.

4 Spoon the frittata mixture almost to the top of each hole of the prepared muffin pan. Top with cherry tomatoes.

5 Cook for 20 minutes, until the tops turn golden brown and the frittatas start to pull away from the sides of the pan.

6 Eat cold or reheat in the microwave for 15–20 seconds on high. Store in an airtight container in the fridge.

TIPS
*Check buying tips (see page 25).

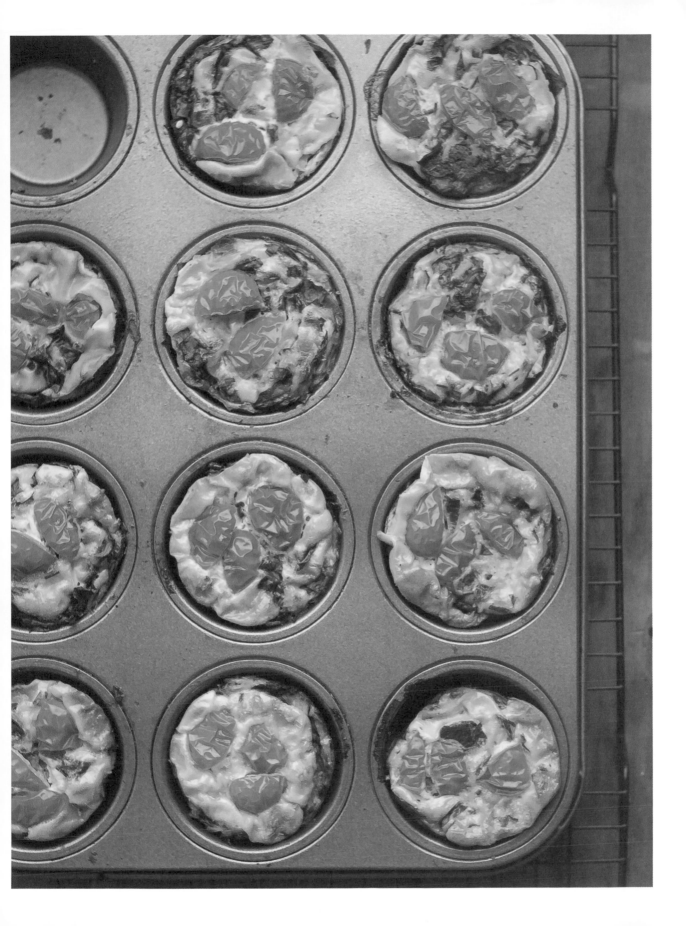

Sweet Red Pepper Soup

PREP TIME: 10 minutes COOK TIME: 40 minutes
SERVES: 4

LF GFO DF EF NF SF

2 red bell peppers, seeded and cut
　into strips
2 large (8½oz/240g) carrots, peeled
　and cut into bite-sized pieces
2 medium (8½oz/240g) parsnips,
　peeled and cut into bite-sized
　pieces
1 tablespoon neutral oil (e.g. canola,
　grapeseed, safflower, sunflower)
A few grinds of salt and pepper
4 cups low-FODMAP chicken or
　vegetable stock* (GF if needed)
1 (15oz/400g) can plain crushed/
　chopped tomatoes
1 tablespoon garlic-infused oil*
2 teaspoons paprika
A few grinds of salt and pepper, to
　taste
8 slices low-FODMAP or gluten-free
　bread,* to serve
3 tablespoons finely chopped parsley,
　to garnish (optional)

This creamy, sweet soup combines rich tomato flavors with the sweetness of roasted red bell pepper, carrot, and parsnip.

1 Preheat oven to 400°F. Place the bell peppers, carrot, and parsnip on a baking sheet. Drizzle with oil and season with salt and pepper. Toss so the veggies are well coated.

2 Roast in the oven for 20–25 minutes, until golden and soft. Toss once during cooking.

3 Once the veggies are cooked, transfer them to a blender or a large saucepan. Add half of the stock and the tomatoes. Blend until smooth using the blender or an immersion blender.

4 Pour the soup into a large saucepan and place over medium heat. Stir in the other half of the stock, the oil, and paprika, and season with salt and pepper. Allow the soup to heat through.

5 Heat the bread in the oven for 5 minutes, until warm.

6 Sprinkle the soup with parsley, if using, and serve with the bread.

TIPS
*Check buying tips (see pages 25–26).

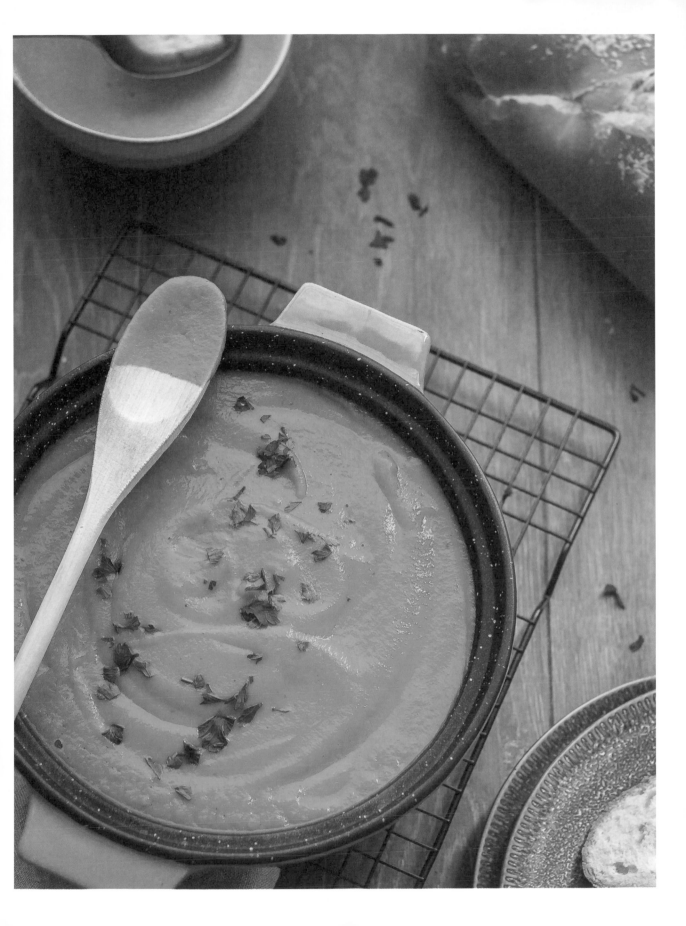

Instant Noodle Bowl

PREP TIME: 15 minutes COOK TIME: 12 minutes
SERVES: 1

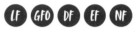

¼ cup (1oz/40g) diced carrot

1 ounce (35g) thin rice noodles or rice vermicelli

½ cup (1oz/30g) shredded bok choy, washed

½ cup (2½oz/70g) diced cooked chicken or firm tofu

2 tablespoons fresh or frozen corn

2 tablespoons finely chopped scallions (green leaves only)

1 teaspoon soy sauce (GF if needed)

½ teaspoon chile puree*

¼ teaspoon crushed ginger*

¼ teaspoon garlic-infused oil*

¼ teaspoon low-FODMAP chicken or vegetable bouillon powder* (GF if needed)

1½ cups boiling water

Squeeze of lemon or lime juice

Sprinkle of fresh cilantro

Most instant noodle cups are high FODMAP so I decided to make my own! The hardest part of this recipe is finding low-FODMAP bouillon powder, so make sure you check your low-FODMAP app for options.

1 Cook the carrot in the microwave for 1 minute 30 seconds on high, then drain.

2 Place the carrot, noodles, bok choy, chicken or tofu, corn, scallions, soy sauce, chile puree, ginger, oil, and bouillon powder in a bowl or lunch container.

3 Ten minutes before you are ready to eat, add the boiling water (make sure the noodles are fully immersed) and cover. Allow to sit for 10 minutes. The noodles should be just cooked; if they aren't, microwave them for 1 minute.

4 Season with a squeeze of lemon or lime juice and a sprinkle of fresh cilantro. Mix well before eating.

TIPS
*Check buying tips (see pages 25–26).

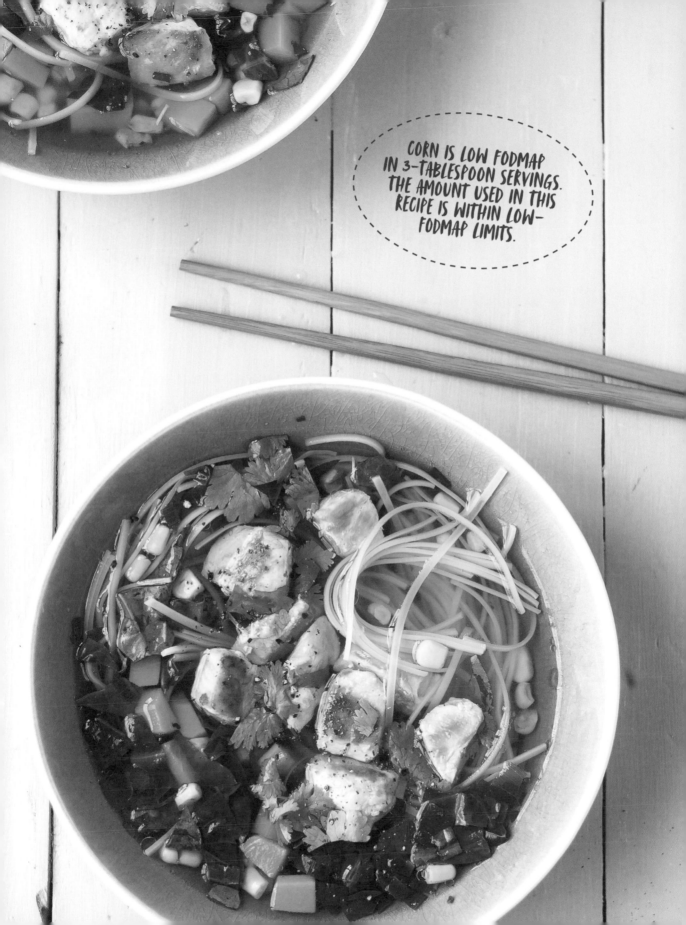

CORN IS LOW FODMAP IN 3-TABLESPOON SERVINGS. THE AMOUNT USED IN THIS RECIPE IS WITHIN LOW-FODMAP LIMITS.

Easy Sandwich Ideas

These simple low-FODMAP sandwiches make delicious lunchbox fillers.

EGG SALAD
PREP TIME: 15 minutes
SERVES: 1

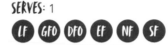

2 eggs
½ teaspoon Dijon mustard*
1 tablespoon chopped fresh chives
½ tablespoon chopped fresh dill
1 tablespoon mayonnaise
A few grinds of salt and pepper, to taste
1 teaspoon dairy-free spread or butter
2 slices low-FODMAP or gluten-free bread*
1 tablespoon alfalfa sprouts

1   Hard-boil the eggs (see page 66). Peel, then mash them with the mustard, chives, dill, and mayonnaise. Season generously with salt and pepper.

2   Butter the low-FODMAP bread, spread one slice with mashed egg, and top with sprouts. Place the other slice of bread on top.

BARBECUE CHICKEN SALAD
PREP TIME: 5 minutes
SERVES: 1

1 teaspoon dairy-free spread or butter
2 slices low-FODMAP or gluten-free bread*
½ cup shredded lettuce (e.g. butter, iceberg, red leaf)
¼ cup (1oz/30g) shredded cooked chicken
2 teaspoon Smoky Barbecue Sauce (see recipe on page 210)
1 tablespoon finely sliced scallions (green leaves only)
A few grinds of salt and pepper, to taste

1   Butter the low-FODMAP bread, place the lettuce on one slice and top with chicken, Smoky Barbecue Sauce, and scallions. Season with salt and pepper. Place the other slice of bread on top.

TIPS
*Check buying tips (see page 26).

CONTINUED ON PAGE 93

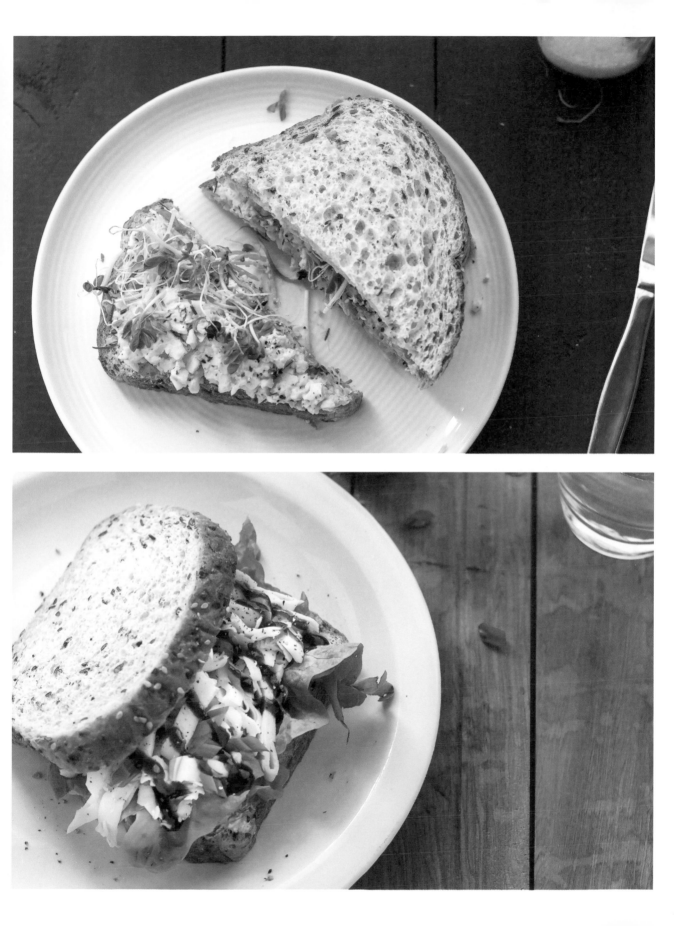

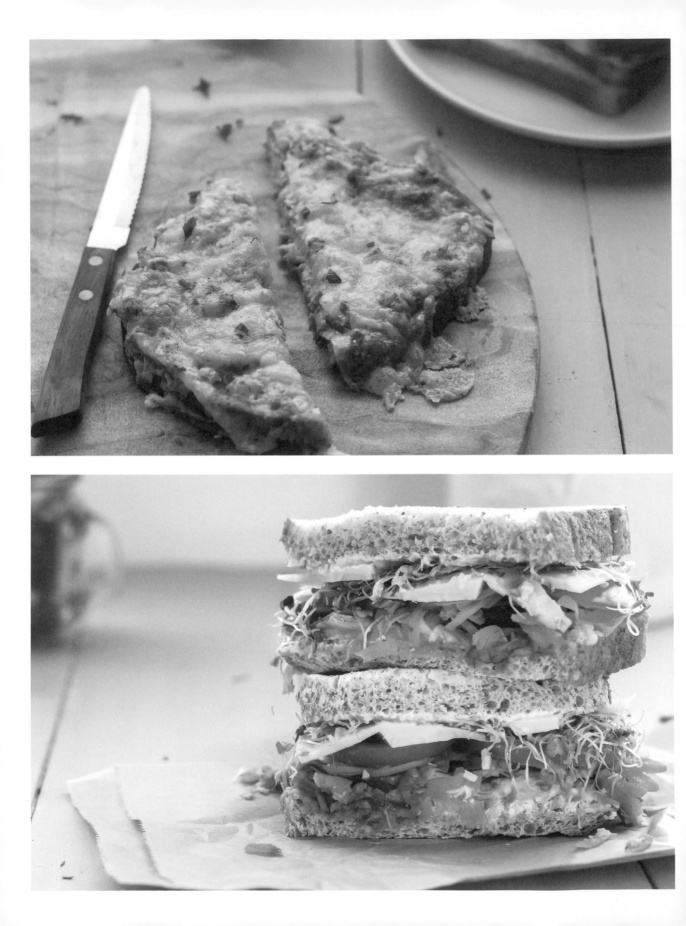

CHEESY TUNA MELT
PREP TIME: 5 minutes **COOK TIME:** 5 minutes
SERVES: 1

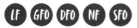

3 ounces (95g) canned tuna in spring water

2 tablespoons mayonnaise

1 teaspoon lemon juice

Sprinkle of paprika

1 tablespoon finely chopped fresh flat-leaf parsley

2 tablespoons finely chopped scallions (green leaves only)

A few grinds of salt and pepper, to taste

2 slices low-FODMAP or gluten-free bread*

4 thin slices (1½oz/40g) Colby, Cheddar, or vegan cheese*

1 Preheat broiler or grill to 400°F.

2 Drain the tuna and mix with the mayonnaise, lemon juice, paprika, parsley, and scallions. Season with salt and pepper.

3 Toast the bread. Spread the mixture on both slices of toast and top with cheese.

4 Place the toast on an oven tray and broil until the cheese is golden.

EASY SALAD & HUMMUS SANDWICH
PREP TIME: 10 minutes
SERVES: 1

2 tablespoons Traditional Hummus (see recipe on page 210)

2 slices low-FODMAP or gluten-free bread*

2 slices Colby, Cheddar, or vegan cheese*

¼ cup shredded lettuce (e.g. butter, iceberg, red leaf)

4 slices canned beets, drained and patted dry

½ tomato, sliced

½ medium carrot, peeled and grated

1 tablespoon alfalfa sprouts

1 Spread the hummus on both slices of bread. Top one slice with the cheese, lettuce, beets, tomato, carrot, and sprouts. Place the other slice of bread on top.

Fresh Spring Rolls with Satay Dipping Sauce

PREP TIME: 45 minutes
SERVES: 4

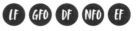

SATAY SAUCE

4 tablespoons sunflower seed butter
    or peanut butter
2 teaspoons Sweet Chile Sauce (see
    recipe on page 214)
4 teaspoons brown sugar
1 teaspoon garlic-infused oil*
2 teaspoons soy sauce (GF if needed)
2 teaspoons lemon juice

SPRING ROLLS

12 rice paper wrappers
1 large (4oz/120g) carrot, peeled and
    julienned
1 red bell pepper, seeded and
    julienned
1 small cucumber, peeled and
    julienned
½ cup (1½oz/45g) shredded red
    cabbage
2 cups (9oz/250g) shredded cooked
    chicken
1 cup chopped fresh cilantro, basil,
    and mint
2 cups shredded lettuce (e.g. butter,
    iceberg, red leaf)
½ teaspoon sesame seeds (optional)

TIPS

To store the rolls, wrap them
individually in plastic wrap (to stop
them from drying out and sticking)
and place in a plastic container.
Store for 2–3 days in the fridge.

*Check buying tips (see page 25).

There is something just so delicious about dipping a rice roll into a sticky satay sauce! These are perfect for lunch or a light dinner.

1 Mix the satay sauce ingredients together in a small bowl until the sauce becomes smooth. If you have trouble mixing the ingredients, heat in the microwave for 20 seconds.

2 Fill a large bowl with warm water. Dip one rice paper wrapper into the water until you feel it start to soften (15–20 seconds). Place the wrapper on a damp tea towel.

3 On the bottom third of the wrapper, place some carrot, bell pepper, cucumber, and a little red cabbage. Add a small layer of chicken, herbs, and lettuce. Try not to overstuff the roll, otherwise things will get messy!

4 Roll it up: fold the two small sides up (like a burrito), then gently pull the bottom of the roll up and roll over the filling (tuck the filling in using your hands). Repeat with the remaining wrappers and fillings.

5 Sprinkle with sesame seeds (if using) and serve with the satay sauce.

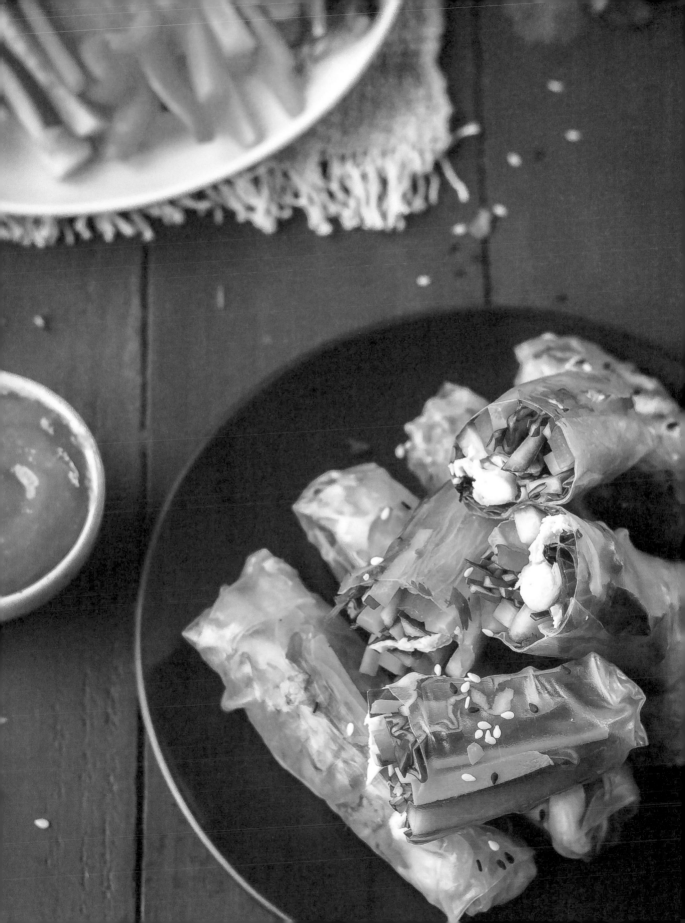

Tasty Egg Wraps

PREP TIME: 10 minutes COOK TIME: 10 minutes
SERVES: 1

LF GF DFO NF SFO

BASIC EGG WRAP

1½ tablespoons low-FODMAP milk*
½ tablespoon gluten-free all-purpose
    flour*
2 large eggs
A few grinds of salt and pepper
Drizzle of neutral oil (e.g. canola,
    grapeseed, safflower, sunflower)

SAUTÉED VEGGIE FILLING

½ cup (1oz/40g) thinly sliced eggplant
½ red bell pepper, cut into strips
1 medium (2oz/60g) carrot, peeled
    and julienned
½ cup (2oz/65g) chopped zucchini
Drizzle of neutral oil (e.g. canola,
    grapeseed, safflower, sunflower)
A few grinds of salt and pepper, to
    taste
Sprinkle of paprika
Zesty Lemon Aïoli (see recipe on page
    212), to serve

HAM & MUSTARD FILLING

1 teaspoon Dijon mustard*
1½ ounces (40g) sliced ham*
Handful of baby spinach, roughly
    chopped

These make a great low-FODMAP alternative to wheat-based wraps. They are yummy warm or cold and you can fill them with a variety of fillings. Here are two of my favorites to get you started.

1 Place a medium frying pan over medium–low heat. Mix together the milk and flour in a medium bowl. Once smooth, whisk in the eggs until the mixture is evenly yellow. Season with salt and pepper.

2 Grease the pan with the oil. Pour the egg mixture into the pan and tip the pan in a circular motion until it is evenly spread over the base. Cook for about 1 minute, until the edges start to lift. Using a spatula, gently flip the wrap and cook for another 30 seconds or so, until golden.

3 To make the sautéed veggie filling, sauté the veggies in a little oil over medium–high heat until the eggplant is golden brown. Season with salt and pepper and a sprinkle of paprika. Spread the filling over the egg wrap and add a drizzle of Zesty Lemon Aïoli. Roll up to serve.

4 To make the ham and mustard filling, spread the mustard on the egg wrap and top with ham and spinach. Roll up to serve.

TIPS
*Check buying tips (see pages
25–27).

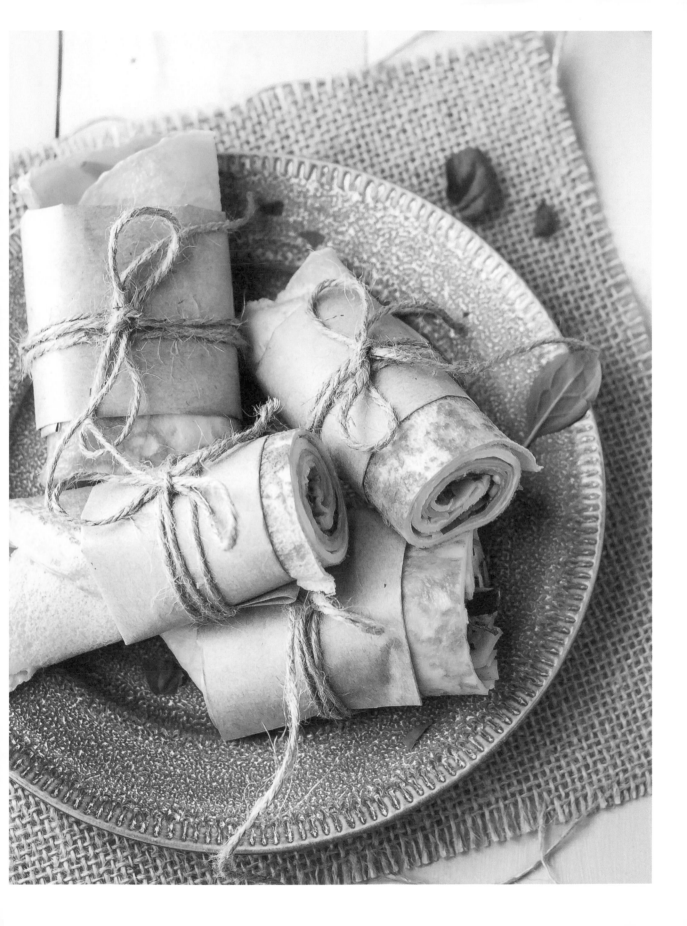

Sweet Orange Chicken Wings

PREP TIME: 5 minutes COOK TIME: 50 minutes
SERVES: 5

LF GFO DF EF NF

2 pounds (1kg) chicken wings

1 tablespoons neutral oil (e.g. canola, grapeseed, safflower, sunflower)

A few grinds of salt and pepper

3 teaspoons sesame seeds

2 tablespoons chopped fresh cilantro, to garnish (optional)

SWEET ORANGE SAUCE

1½ teaspoons orange zest

¼ cup (60ml) freshly squeezed orange juice

¼ cup (60ml) low-FODMAP chicken stock* (GF if needed)

2 teaspoons corn starch (GF if needed), dissolved in warm water

1 tablespoons soy sauce (GF if needed)

2 tablespoons brown sugar

TIPS

If you don't have low-FODMAP chicken stock, you can use the juices from the pan.

*Check buying tips (see page 26).

The combination of freshly squeezed orange juice, soy sauce, and sesame seeds creates finger-licking-good chicken wings. These make the perfect weekend lunch or plate to take to a barbecue.

1 Preheat oven to 400°F. Line a large roasting pan with parchment paper.

2 Place the chicken wings in a large bowl and toss them with the oil and a few grinds of salt and black pepper.

3 Arrange the chicken wings in a single layer in the prepared roasting pan. Bake for 45–50 minutes, turning the chicken wings halfway through, until golden and the juices run clear.

4 Toast the sesame seeds in a small frying pan over medium heat (no oil needed). Stir them constantly, otherwise they will burn. Remove once they start to brown and tip out onto a plate.

5 To make the sweet orange sauce, place the orange zest and juice in a small saucepan. Add the chicken stock, corn starch mixture, soy sauce, and brown sugar and stir well. Heat the sauce over a low heat, stirring occasionally, until thick.

6 Dip the chicken wings in the sauce. Place on a plate and sprinkle with sesame seeds. Garnish with fresh cilantro, if desired. This dish is a bit messy! I would recommend serving it with a bowl of lemon water and a hand towel so your guests can clean their fingers.

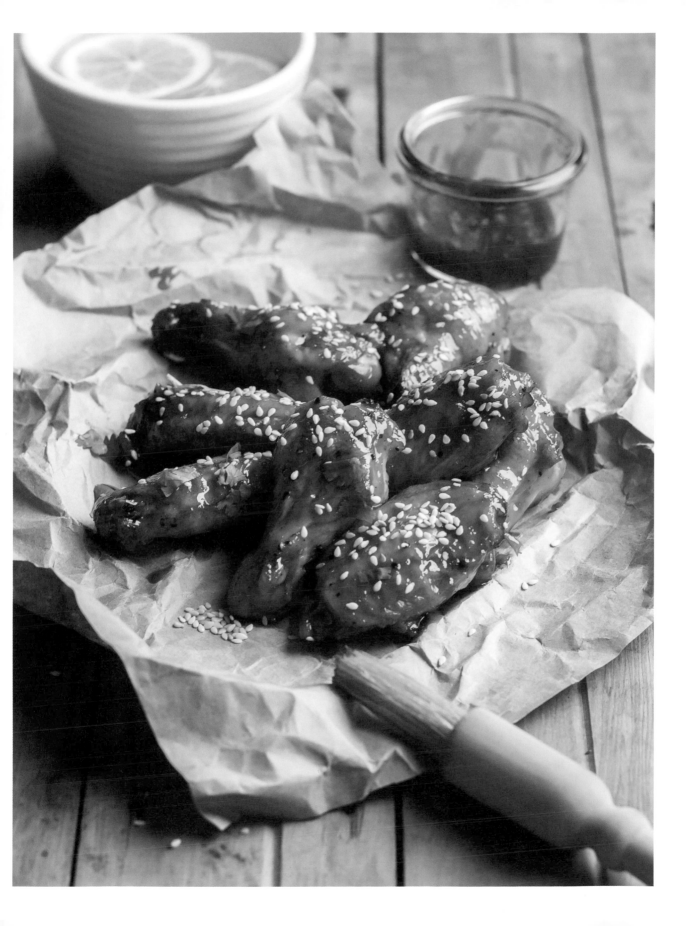

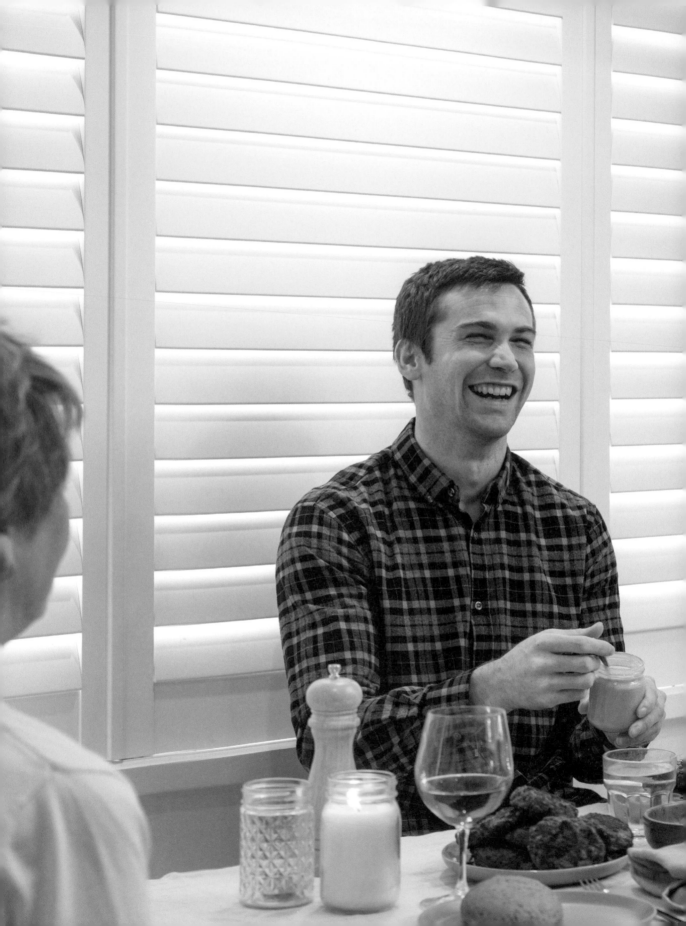

DINNER

There's nothing better than gathering around the table to share good food and laughter with friends and family.

Sticky Chinese Chicken Bake

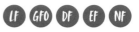

1¼ pounds (600g) boneless chicken thighs

2½ cups (625ml) low-FODMAP chicken stock* (GF if needed)

2 large (8½oz/240g) carrots, peeled and diced

2 cups (8½oz/240g) peeled and diced kabocha squash/Japanese pumpkin

1¼ cups long-grain white rice or basmati rice

1 cup (2½oz/80g) chopped leeks (green leaves only)

1 tablespoon neutral oil (e.g. canola, grapeseed, safflower, sunflower)

1½ cups (6oz/180g) chopped green beans

A few grinds of black pepper, to taste

3 tablespoons roughly chopped fresh cilantro, to garnish

STICKY MARINADE

1 teaspoon lemon zest

2 tablespoons freshly squeezed lemon juice

4 tablespoons soy sauce (GF if needed)

4 tablespoons pure maple syrup

1 tablespoon garlic-infused oil

1 teaspoon crushed ginger*

TIPS

*Check buying tips (see pages 25–26).

This delicious bake is sure to be a hit with the whole family!

1 Preheat oven to 375°F. Grease a deep baking dish or roasting pan that's about 2½ inches deep.

2 Mix the marinade ingredients together and pour over the chicken thighs. Leave to marinate for at least 5 minutes, ideally an hour.

3 Pour the stock into a microwave-proof bowl and heat until hot (1–2 minutes on high).

4 Put the carrot and squash in a microwave-proof bowl. Add 3 tablespoons of water and cook in the microwave for 3–4 minutes on high until they start to soften. Drain.

5 Place the carrot, pumpkin, rice, leeks, and hot stock in the baking dish. Remove the chicken from the marinade and reserve 3 tablespoons of marinade. Stir the remaining marinade into the rice mixture. Cover tightly with foil and bake for 30–40 minutes, until the rice is tender and sticky. Stir after 20 minutes.

6 Add the oil to a frying pan and sear the chicken thighs over medium–high heat for 4 minutes on each side, until golden brown (but not cooked through). Place on an oven tray and baste with half of the reserved marinade. Bake for 10 minutes, baste again, and cook for another 5 minutes. Remove from the oven once the chicken is cooked through (juices should run clear; cook for longer if using whole chicken thighs).

7 Five minutes before serving, blanch the green beans, then drain. Mix the green beans and chicken pan juices through the rice. Top with the chicken and season with black pepper. Garnish with fresh cilantro.

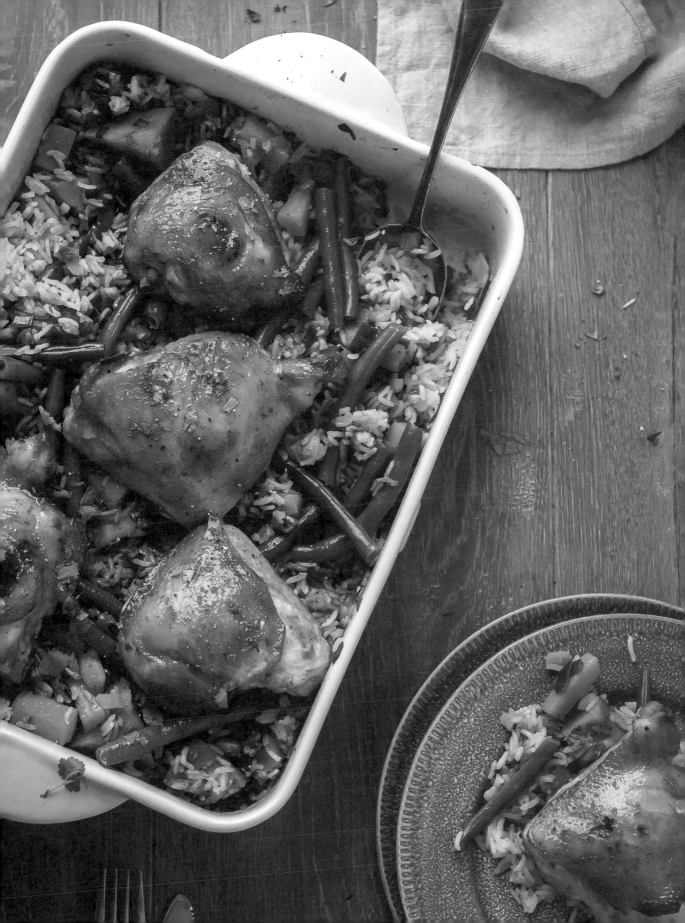

Roast Chicken with Homemade Gravy

PREP TIME: 20 minutes **COOK TIME**: 1 hour 40 minutes
SERVES: 4 (plus leftovers)

LF GFO DF EF NF SF

1 (3lb/1.3kg) whole chicken*
Drizzle of olive oil
A few grinds of salt and pepper
1 lemon
Handful of fresh rosemary and thyme
2 large (8½oz/240g) carrots, peeled
　and cut into large pieces
2 medium (8½oz/240g) parsnips,
　peeled and cut into large pieces
1¼ pounds (600g) potatoes, peeled
　and cut into large pieces
1½ cups (6oz/180g) chopped green
　beans
2 cups (6oz/180g) chopped broccoli
Chopped fresh herbs, to garnish

GRAVY

Pan juices from the roast (about
　½ cup/125ml)
1 cup (250ml) low-FODMAP chicken
　stock* (GF if needed)
1 tablespoon corn starch (GF if
　needed)
2 tablespoons warm water
2 tablespoons roughly chopped fresh
　parsley

Roast chicken is a favorite for Sunday night family dinners. This homey, low-FODMAP meal is super easy, and even includes homemade gravy. If you are feeling like a kitchen superhero, whip up a batch of Crunchy Herb Stuffing (see recipe on page 194) to serve on the side.

1 Preheat oven to 375°F. Place the chicken in a roasting pan, drizzle with olive oil, then season with salt and pepper. Pierce the lemon and place it inside the chicken cavity along with the fresh herbs.

2 Cook the chicken in the oven for 1½ hours (or according to instructions). The chicken is cooked once the juices run clear. Remove the chicken from the pan (keep ½ cup of the juices in the pan) and allow to rest for 10 minutes before carving.

3 In a roasting pan, toss the carrot, parsnip, and potato with a drizzle of olive oil. Once the chicken has cooked for 40 minutes, place the veggies in the oven and cook until golden brown.

4 To make the gravy, place the chicken roasting pan on the stovetop over medium–high heat. Add the stock and scrape the brown bits off the bottom of the pan until they dissolve. Then dissolve the corn starch in the warm water and add to the gravy. Allow to thicken, stirring occasionally. Stir the parsley into the gravy.

5 Just before serving, blanch the green beans and broccoli in boiling water for 2–3 minutes, until tender.

6 Serve the chicken with the roasted veggies, broccoli, green beans, and gravy. Garnish with chopped fresh herbs.

TIPS
*Check buying tips (see page 26).

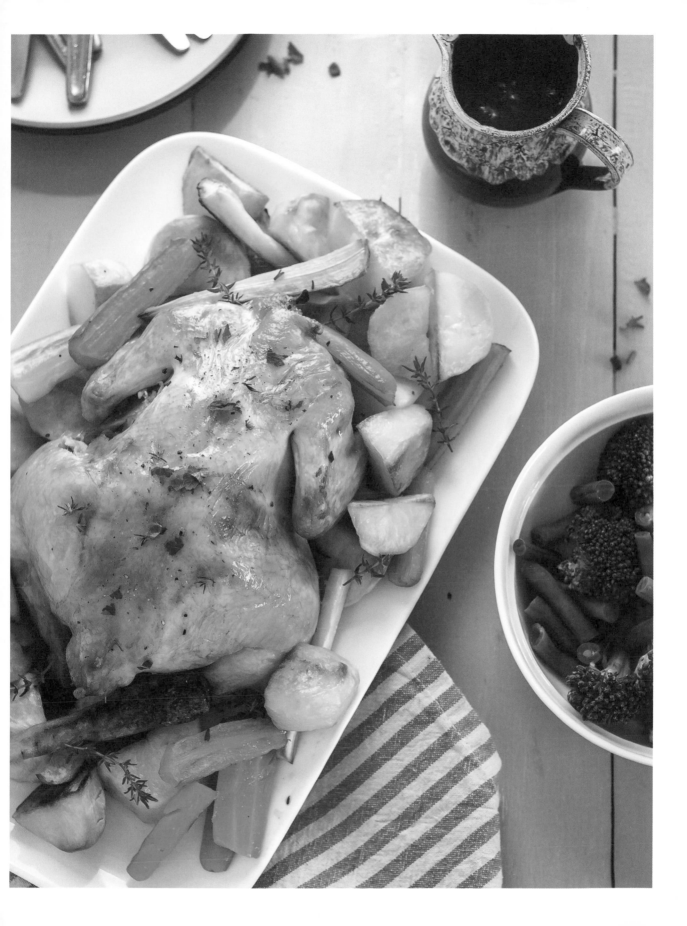

Homemade Butter Chicken

LF GFO DF EF NF SF

1¼ cups long-grain white rice or
  basmati rice
1½ teaspoons neutral oil (e.g. canola,
  grapeseed, safflower, sunflower)
1 pound (450g) boneless chicken
  thighs (skin and fat removed), diced
2 large (8½oz/240g) carrots, peeled
  and diced
1½ teaspoons crushed ginger*
½ teaspoon crushed red pepper/
  pureed red chile*
2 cups (500ml) low-FODMAP chicken
  stock* (GF if needed)
6 tablespoons tomato paste
1 cup (250ml) canned coconut milk*
4 cups (4oz/120g) spinach
A few grinds of salt and black pepper,
  to taste
Pinch of sugar, to taste (optional)
4 tablespoons roughly chopped fresh
  cilantro

SPICE MIX

¾ teaspoon mild curry powder*
½ teaspoon garam masala
½ teaspoon ground turmeric
½ teaspoon salt
¼ teaspoon fennel seeds
¼ teaspoon mustard seeds
¼ teaspoon ground coriander

TIPS

*Check buying tips (see pages
25–27).

I love creating fake-out! This butter chicken won't be quite as authentic as the one from your local Indian take-out, but it is pretty darn tasty.

1 Cook the rice according to package instructions.

2 Heat the oil in a large frying pan over medium–high heat. Fry the chicken until golden.

3 While you wait, place the spice mix ingredients in a small container.

4 Once the chicken is cooked, add the carrot, ginger, chile, and spice mix to the pan. Fry for 1 minute, until fragrant, then mix in the chicken stock, tomato paste (measure it carefully), and coconut milk. Turn down the heat and simmer for about 20 minutes, then add the spinach. Simmer for another 5 minutes. Taste and season with salt and pepper and a pinch of sugar, if needed.

5 Once the curry reaches your desired thickness, serve over the rice and sprinkle with fresh cilantro.

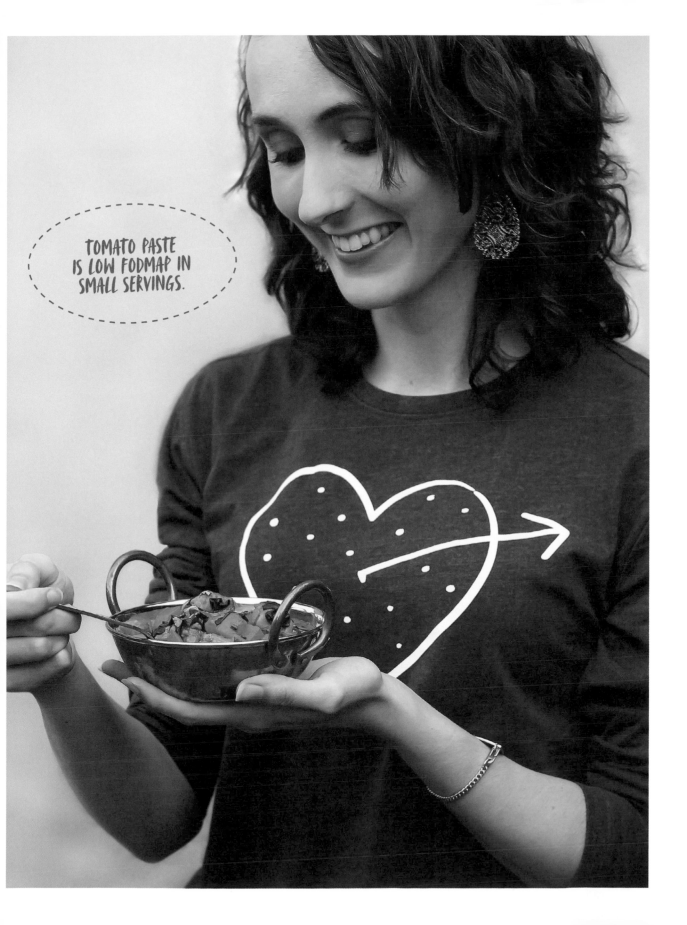

Chicken & Roasted Veggie Pasta in Red Wine Sauce

PREP TIME: 10 minutes **COOK TIME:** 30 minutes
SERVES: 4

(LF) (GF) (DF) (EF) (NF) (SF)

2 large (8½oz/240g) carrots, peeled and cut into small pieces

3 cups (8½oz/240g) cubed eggplant

Drizzle of olive oil

A few grinds of salt and pepper

1 pound (450g) chicken breast, cut into cubes

½ recipe Red Wine & Tomato Pasta Sauce (see recipe on page 110)

3 cups (3oz/90g) roughly chopped spinach

10 ounces (280g) gluten-free spaghetti*

2 tablespoons chopped flat-leaf parsley

This saucy number is sure to be a crowd pleaser and is a great way to use my homemade Red Wine & Tomato Pasta Sauce.

1 Preheat oven to 375°F. Place the carrot and eggplant on a baking sheet, drizzle with olive oil, and season well with salt and pepper. Roast for 20–30 minutes, turning once, until golden and soft.

2 While the veggies roast, fry the chicken with a drizzle of oil in a large frying pan over medium–high heat for 4–5 minutes, until golden brown and cooked through. Turn the heat down to low and add the pasta sauce and spinach. Allow to heat through.

3 Cook the spaghetti according to package instructions. Drain, and then toss through the sauce along with the roasted veggies. Season with salt and pepper and garnish with parsley.

TIPS
*Check buying tips (see page 25).

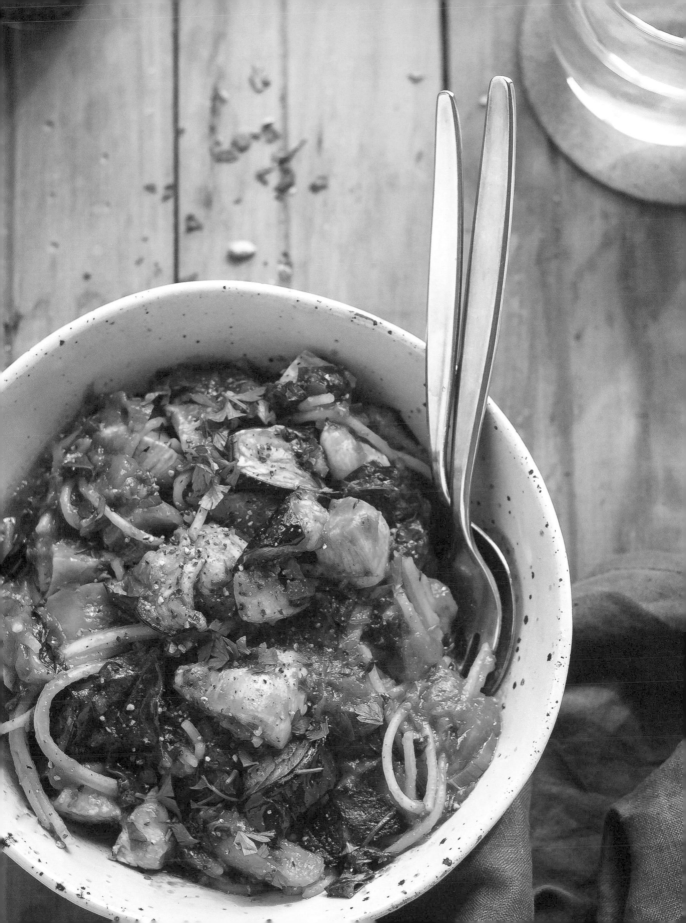

Red Wine & Tomato Pasta Sauce

PREP TIME: 10 minutes COOK TIME: 50 minutes
SERVES: 8

(LF) (GFO) (DF) (EF) (NF) (SF)

2 tablespoons garlic-infused oil*

1 tablespoon olive oil

1 cup (2½oz/80g) finely chopped leeks
   (green leaves only)

1 (28oz/800g) can plain crushed/
   chopped tomatoes

¼ cup (60ml) red wine

4 tablespoons tomato paste

1 cup (250ml) low-FODMAP chicken or
   vegetable stock* (GF if needed)

1½ teaspoons white sugar

2 teaspoons dried oregano

1½ teaspoons dried thyme

¾ teaspoon dried rosemary

A few grinds of salt and pepper, to
   taste

Splash of Worcestershire sauce* (GF if
   needed; optional)

Handful of fresh herbs (optional)

Looking for a tasty low-FODMAP pasta sauce? This one is ideal! Cook a double batch and freeze or bottle the leftover sauce for easy 15-minute meals. It's perfect for shepherd's pie, lasagna, spaghetti Bolognese, or pasta dishes. Just remember to use only half a cup per serving (avoid using larger serving sizes as they may be higher in FODMAPs).

1 Heat the garlic-infused oil and olive oil in a large saucepan over medium–high heat. Fry the leeks until fragrant.

2 Stir in the tomatoes, red wine, tomato paste, stock, sugar, and dried herbs. Season generously with salt and pepper.

3 Turn down the heat to medium–low. Simmer for 35–40 minutes, stirring occasionally. Taste and add more seasonings or salt and pepper as needed. If you want to add more depth of flavor to your sauce, try adding a splash of Worcestershire sauce. Or boost the flavor even further by adding a handful of fresh herbs before serving.

TIPS

This pasta sauce will keep for
5 days in the fridge, for 3 months
in the freezer, or you can bottle it
and store it safely for at least
6 months in the pantry
(unopened).

*Check buying tips (see pages
25–26).

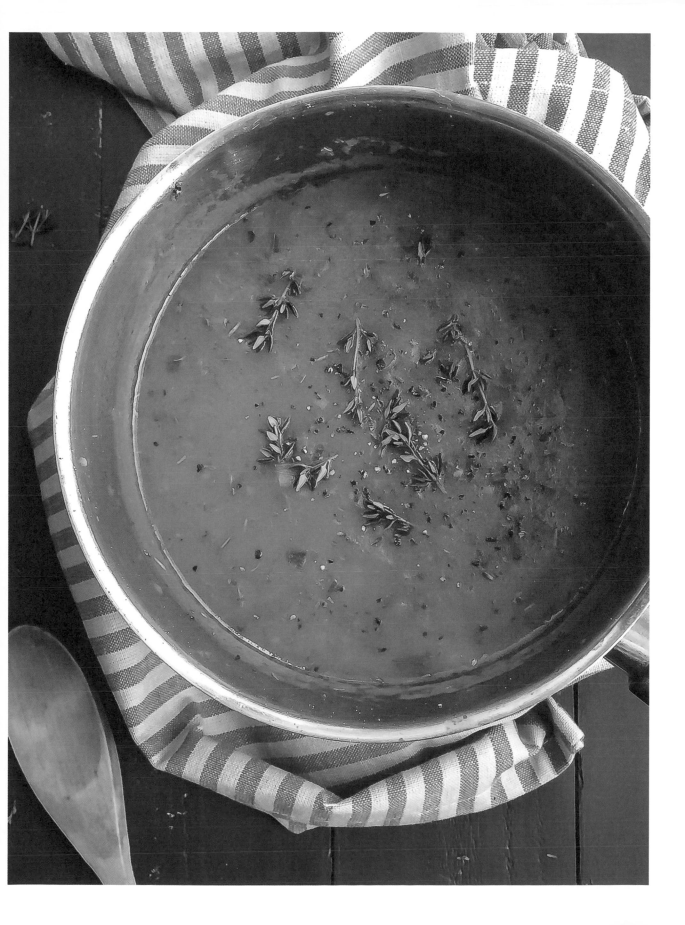

Basic Beef Burgers with Maple Mustard Dressing

PREP TIME: 20 minutes **COOK TIME:** 20 minutes
SERVES: 4

LF **GFO** **DF** **NF** **SFO**

BEEF PATTIES

1½ pounds (650g) lean ground beef

½ cup gluten-free breadcrumbs*

¼ cup finely chopped scallions (green
    leaves only)

¼ cup chopped fresh parsley

2 tablespoons tomato paste

1 tablespoon soy sauce (GF if needed)

1 teaspoon dried oregano

½ teaspoon dried thyme

¼ teaspoon Chinese five spice*

1 large egg, beaten

A few grinds of salt and pepper

1 tablespoon olive oil, for cooking

TO SERVE

4 low-FODMAP or gluten-free burger
    buns*

4 large lettuce leaves or 2 cups small
    leaves

2 medium tomatoes, sliced

Maple Mustard Dressing (see recipe
    on page 213)

I love a good burger! The juiciness of the beef patty combined with crisp lettuce and tomato, topped off with a drizzle of Maple Mustard Dressing, is just heaven. Break these burgers out at your next barbecue or enjoy them as an easy Friday-night meal.

1 Place all the beef patty ingredients except the olive oil in a large bowl. Mix together with your hands until thoroughly combined. Divide evenly into patties (two patties per person) that are no thicker than ½ inch thick.

2 Heat the oil in a large frying pan over medium–low heat and cook the patties for 6–7 minutes on each side, until browned and cooked through. Transfer the patties to a plate and keep warm. You might need to cook them in two batches. You can also cook them on the barbecue.

3 Place the beef patties on the burger buns, then add lettuce leaves, tomato, and a drizzle of Maple Mustard Dressing.

TIPS

To make this recipe soy free, replace the soy sauce and Chinese five spice with 1 tablespoon of Worcestershire sauce.

*Check buying tips (see pages 25–26).

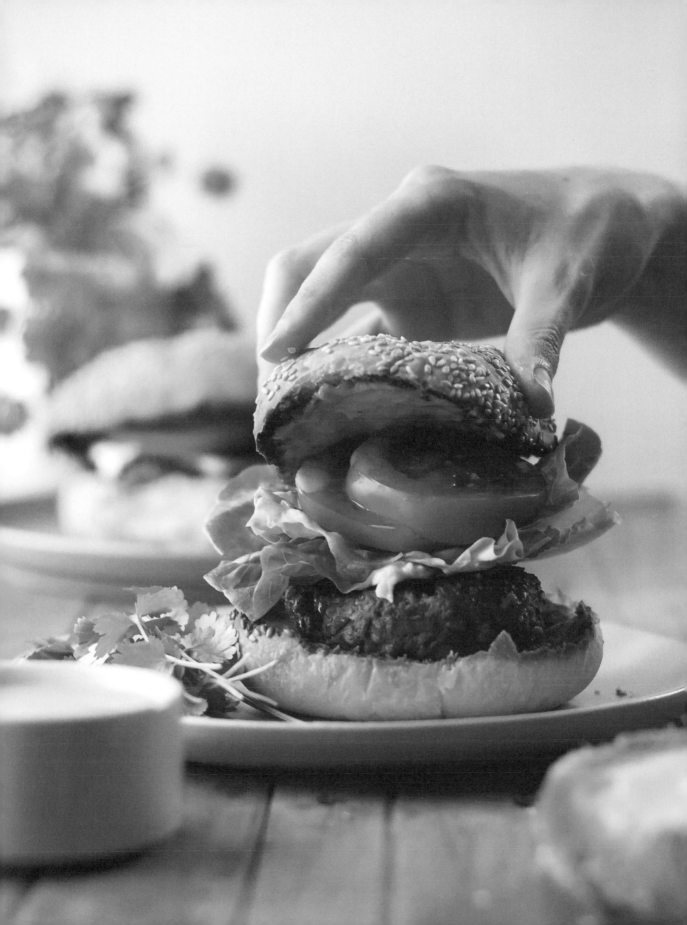

Beef Enchiladas

ENCHILADA SAUCE

1 (15oz/400g) can plain crushed/
    chopped tomatoes, pureed
½ cup (125ml) low-FODMAP chicken
    stock* (GF if needed)
2 tablespoons tomato paste
4 teaspoons paprika
2 teaspoons dried oregano
2 teaspoons ground cumin
1½ teaspoons ground coriander
1 teaspoon white sugar
¼ teaspoon chile powder* (or to taste)
¼ teaspoon each of salt and black
    pepper
1 tablespoon corn starch (GF if needed)

ENCHILADAS

8 corn tortillas (GF if needed)
3 teaspoons garlic-infused oil*
1 pound (450g) lean ground beef
1 cup (2½oz/80g) chopped leeks
    (green leaves only)
1 (15oz/400g) can lentils, drained and
    rinsed
½ cup (2oz/55g) grated Colby,
    Cheddar, or vegan cheese*
Chopped fresh parsley, to garnish

COLESLAW

2 medium (4oz/120g) carrots
1 cup (3oz/90g) shredded red cabbage
2 cups (5oz/140g) shredded iceberg
    lettuce
Squeeze of lemon juice

TIPS

*Check buying tips (see pages
25–26).

These easy beef enchiladas are always in hot demand in my household and vanish very quickly!

1 To make the sauce, place the pureed tomato in a small saucepan with the other sauce ingredients except the corn starch. Gently simmer over medium–low heat, stirring occasionally, while you cook the beef. Then dissolve the corn starch in a small amount of cold water and mix. Allow to thicken for 1–2 minutes, then taste and add more chile powder, if needed.

2 Warm the tortillas according to package instructions. If you use cold corn tortillas, they will crack and won't wrap nicely.

3 Heat the garlic-infused oil in a large frying pan over medium–high heat. Brown the ground beef, then stir in the leeks and lentils. Reserve ¾ cup of enchilada sauce and mix the rest through the beef. Simmer for 1–2 minutes, then taste. Season with salt and pepper, if needed.

4 Preheat oven to 350°F. Grease a baking dish large enough to snuggly fit all the enchiladas.

5 Place the tortillas in the baking dish so each one forms a U-shape for the filling to go in. Divide the beef mixture evenly among the tortillas, fold the sides on top of the mixture, then roll the tortillas over so the seam is on the bottom. Top with the reserved enchilada sauce and grated cheese. Bake for 15 minutes, or until the cheese is golden brown.

6 While the enchiladas cook, make the coleslaw. Peel and grate the carrots, then toss the ingredients together in a large bowl, with a squeeze of lemon juice.

7 Serve the enchiladas hot with a side of coleslaw. Garnish with parsley.

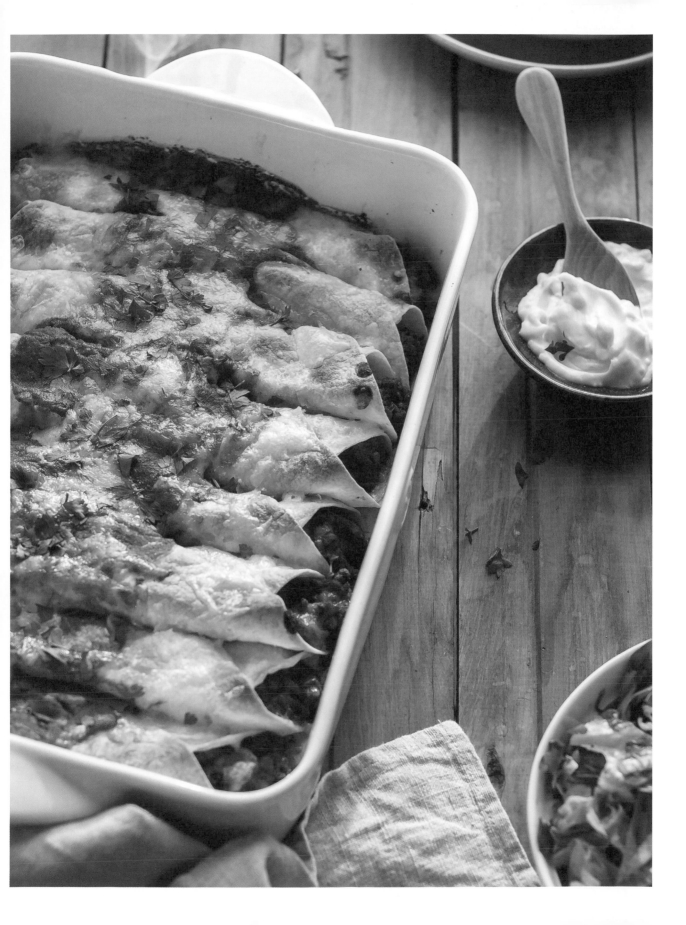

Spicy Beef Lettuce Cups

PREP TIME: 10 minutes COOK TIME: 20 minutes
SERVES: 4

(LF) (GFO) (DF) (EF) (NF)

1¼ cups long-grain white rice or
   basmati rice

1 tablespoon sesame oil

1 pound (450g) lean ground beef

2 teaspoons crushed ginger*

1½ teaspoons crushed red pepper/
   pureed red chile* (or to taste)

2 tablespoons brown sugar

½ tablespoon rice wine vinegar

2 tablespoons soy sauce (GF if
   needed)

A few grinds of black pepper, to taste

1 red bell pepper, cut into large pieces

2 cups (6oz/170g) shredded bok choy

1½ cups (4½oz/135g) shredded red
   cabbage

¼ cup finely sliced scallions (green
   leaves only)

8 small (10oz/290g) iceberg lettuce
   leaves

These spicy beef lettuce cups are my low-FODMAP take on Beef San Choi Bao. You can make them as spicy as you like by either increasing or reducing the amount of crushed red pepper you use in the recipe.

1 Cook the rice according to package instructions.

2 Heat the sesame oil in a large frying pan over medium–high heat. Cook the ground beef for 4–5 minutes, until browned. Turn the heat down to medium. Add the ginger, chile, brown sugar, rice wine vinegar, and soy sauce. Season with black pepper and mix.

3 Add the red bell pepper to the pan and cook for 2 minutes until it starts to soften. Mix in the bok choy, red cabbage, and scallions. Cook for another minute.

4 Serve the spicy beef in the lettuce cups, with the rice.

TIPS
*Check buying tips (see page 25).

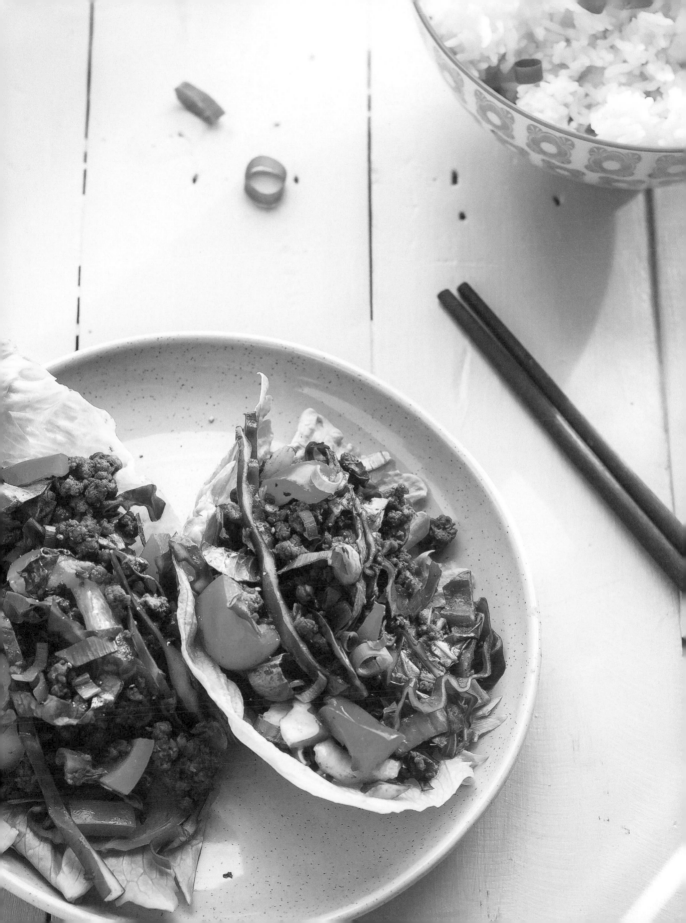

Spaghetti Bolognese

(LF) (GF) (DFO) (EF) (NF) (SF)

1 tablespoon olive oil

1 pound (450g) lean ground beef

1 (15oz/400g) can plain crushed/
chopped tomatoes

3 tablespoons tomato paste

½ cup (1oz/40g) finely chopped leeks
(green leaves only)

4 cups (4oz/20g) roughly chopped
baby spinach

1 teaspoon dried oregano

1 teaspoon dried basil

½ teaspoon dried thyme

A few grinds of salt and pepper, to
taste

10 ounces (280g) gluten-free
spaghetti*

1½ cups (6½oz/190g) chopped green
beans

2 large (8½oz/240g) carrots, peeled
and cut into sticks

½ cup (2oz/55g) grated Cheddar or
vegan cheese* (optional)

Fresh basil, to serve (optional)

This is an easy meal to throw together at the last minute. It is comfort food at its finest and, with the right herbs, you can bring a little bit of Italy right to your table.

1 Heat the olive oil in a large frying pan over medium heat. Cook the ground beef until browned.

2 Add the tomatoes, tomato paste, leeks, spinach, and herbs to the beef. Mix well and simmer over medium–low heat for 20 minutes. Season with salt and pepper.

3 Cook the spaghetti according to package instructions, until soft. Drain the pasta and toss with a drizzle of olive oil.

4 While the spaghetti cooks, blanch the green beans and carrots in a medium saucepan of boiling water for 2–3 minutes, until they are brightly colored and soft.

5 Serve the Bolognese on top of the spaghetti, with a sprinkle of cheese, if using, and the green beans and carrots on the side. Garnish with fresh basil, if desired.

TIPS
*Check buying tips (see pages
25–26).

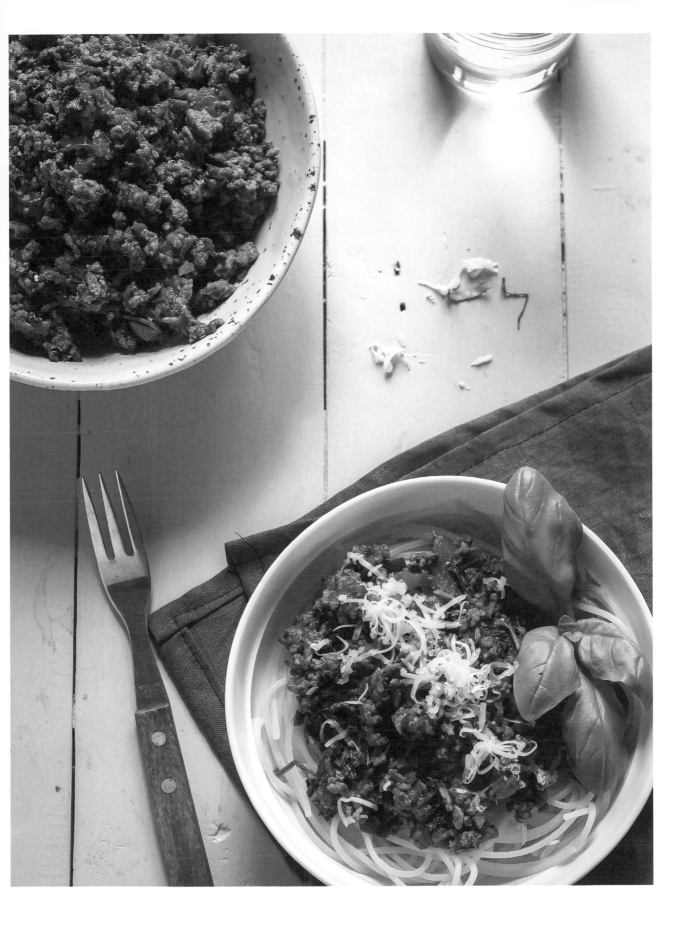

Seared Steak with Smoky Red Pepper Dressing

PREP TIME: 15 minutes **COOK TIME:** 50 minutes
SERVES: 4

(LF) (GF) (DF) (EF) (NF) (SF)

1¼ pounds (600g) potatoes, peeled and cut into large pieces

1 tablespoon olive oil

½ teaspoon Italian mixed herbs (no onion or garlic)

A few grinds of salt and pepper

Drizzle of olive oil

1 pound (450g) beef rump steak, sliced into large steaks

4 cups shredded lettuce (e.g. butter, iceberg, red leaf)

20 cherry tomatoes

1 small cucumber, peeled and sliced

Smoky Red Pepper Dressing (see recipe on page 214), to serve

Chopped fresh parsley, to garnish

This recipe contains one of my favorite dressings of all time: Smoky Red Pepper Dressing! It's smoky and sweet and is the perfect accompaniment for seared steak, salad, or burgers. Round off this meal with a delicious side of crunchy roasted potatoes.

1 Preheat oven to 400°F.

2 Place the potatoes in a roasting pan, drizzle with olive oil, and season with herbs, salt, and pepper. Bake in the oven for 40–50 minutes, until golden and crunchy. Turn once during cooking.

3 Heat a large frying pan over medium–high heat. Add a drizzle of olive oil and sear the steaks for about 4 minutes on each side (this should give you a medium-rare steak) or continue cooking to your preference. Rest them for 5 minutes before serving.

4 Make a salad by tossing together the lettuce, tomato, and cucumber.

5 Serve the seared steak with the salad and crunchy potatoes, then drizzle with Smoky Red Pepper Dressing. Garnish with chopped parsley.

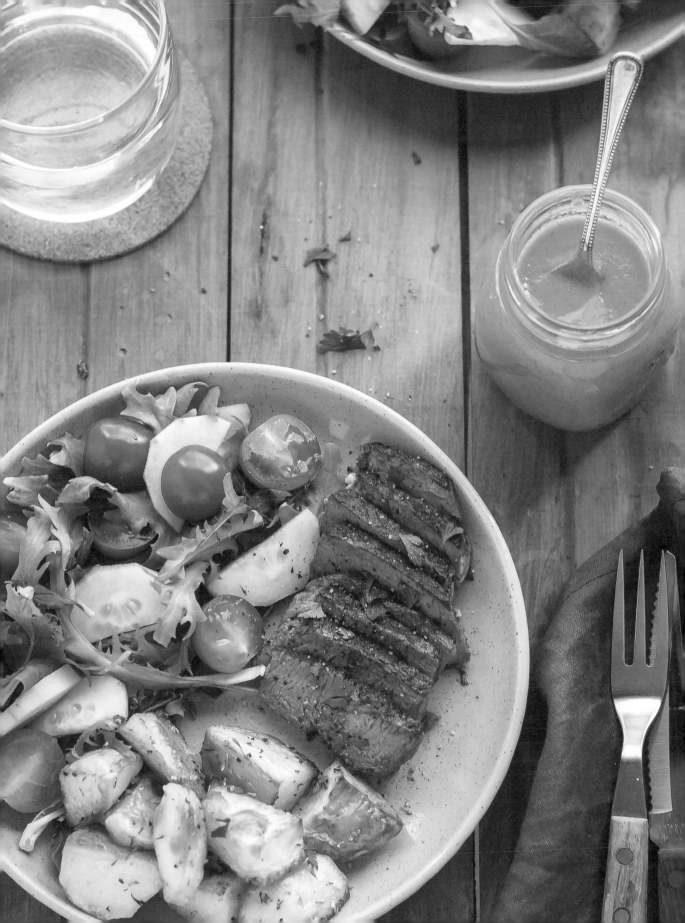

Cumin Lamb & Carrot Pizza with Zesty Lemon Aïoli

PREP TIME: 30 minutes **COOK TIME:** 25 minutes
SERVES: 4

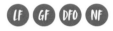

1 red bell pepper, seeded and sliced
   into strips

3 medium (6oz/180g) carrots, peeled
   and cut into bite-sized pieces

1 tablespoon neutral oil (e.g. canola,
   grapeseed, safflower, sunflower)

A few grinds of salt and pepper

7 ounces (200g) canned plain crushed/
   chopped tomatoes

2 gluten-free pizza bases*

1½ teaspoons dried oregano

1 teaspoon cumin seeds

1 cup (1oz/30g) roughly chopped baby
   spinach

1 cup (4oz/115g) grated mozzarella or
   soy-based vegan cheese* (optional)

1 pound (450g) lamb leg steaks

3 tablespoons thinly sliced fresh chives

SIDE SALAD

1 medium (2oz/60g) carrot, peeled
   and grated

3 cups (3oz/90g) finely chopped baby
   spinach

½ cup (4oz/120g) grated zucchini

1 recipe Zesty Lemon Aïoli (see recipe
   on page 212), to serve

A few grinds of salt and pepper

Don't judge this pizza before you try it . . . the flavor combos create a taste sensation. It's sweet, savory, and zesty all at the same time. This recipe is a winner and is well and truly adored by my foodie friends.

1 Preheat oven to 400°F. Place the bell pepper and carrot in a roasting pan, drizzle with oil, and season with salt and pepper. Bake for about 20 minutes, until the carrot softens.

2 While the veggies cook, puree the tomatoes. Cover the pizza bases with pureed tomato and sprinkle evenly with oregano and cumin seeds. Top with spinach and grated cheese, if desired.

3 Once the roasted veggies are cooked, arrange them over the bases. Bake for about 15 minutes, until the bases are golden brown (or according to package instructions).

4 While the pizzas cook, prepare the lamb steaks and make the side salad. Season the lamb by rubbing it with a drizzle of oil, and salt and pepper. Heat a large nonstick frying pan over medium–high heat. Cook the lamb steaks for 3–4 minutes on each side, until medium-rare. Rest them for 4 minutes before slicing them thinly.

5 Toss the salad veggies together in a large bowl, then mix in a large spoonful of Zesty Lemon Aïoli. Season with salt and pepper.

6 Top the pizza with the hot lamb and sprinkle with the chives. Drizzle with Zesty Lemon Aïoli. Serve the salad alongside.

TIPS
*Check buying tips (see page 26).

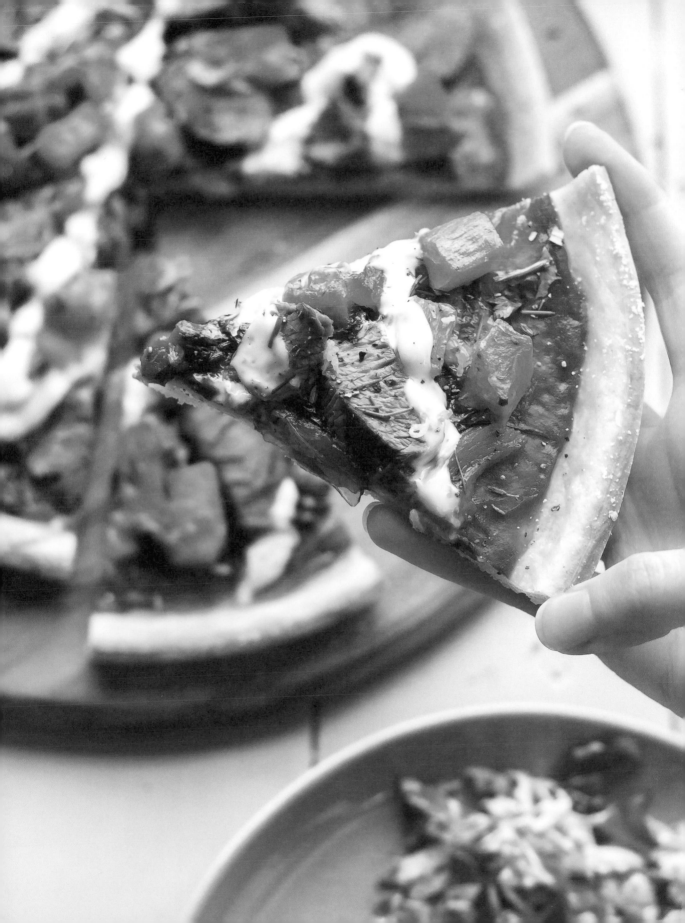

Sticky Pork Ribs

PREP TIME: 30 minutes **COOK TIME**: 2½ hours
SERVES: 6

LF **GFO** **DF** **EF** **NF**

3½ pounds (1.5kg) pork spare ribs
1 tablespoon garlic-infused oil*
1 cup (2½oz/80g) chopped leeks
   (green leaves only)

SPICE RUB

3 teaspoons paprika
1 tablespoon brown sugar
2 teaspoons ground cumin
½ teaspoon salt
1 teaspoon black pepper
Pinch of crushed red pepper*
   (optional)

SAUCE

1 cup (250ml) low-FODMAP chicken
   stock* (GF if needed)
1 cup (250ml) freshly squeezed orange
   juice (3 large oranges)
5 ounces (140g) tomato paste
2 tablespoons soy sauce (GF if
   needed)
2 tablespoons rice wine vinegar
2 teaspoons yellow mustard powder
2 teaspoons Worcestershire sauce*
   (GF if needed)

Sticky, tender, and oh-so-delicious! What's not to love about these slow-roasted pork ribs? Make them for your next barbecue or family dinner. I like to marinate the ribs in the spice rub overnight, but if you are short on time you can skip this step.

1   If cooking immediately, preheat oven to 325°F.

2   Remove the white membrane from the ribs. Pierce the membrane with a sharp knife, slice a strip (to get it started), then peel it off using your hands and a paper towel (the paper towel will help you grip the membrane).

3   Combine the spice rub ingredients in a small bowl. Rub the meat with the spice mixture and leave it for at least 30 minutes (I like to do this the night before). If you are in a rush, just add the spice mixture to the sauce.

4   Heat a large frying pan over medium–high heat. Add the oil and brown the meaty side of the ribs and the leeks for 3–4 minutes. Transfer to a roasting pan.

5   While you fry the pork ribs, make the sauce. In a small saucepan over medium heat, mix together the sauce ingredients (and spice rub mixture, if you haven't already used it) and heat for 3–4 minutes.

6   Pour the sauce over the pork. Cover with foil and bake for 1½ hours, then check if the pork is tender. If it isn't tender, cover it again and continue cooking for another 30 minutes.

TIPS

*Check buying tips (see pages 25–26).

CONTINUED ON PAGE 126

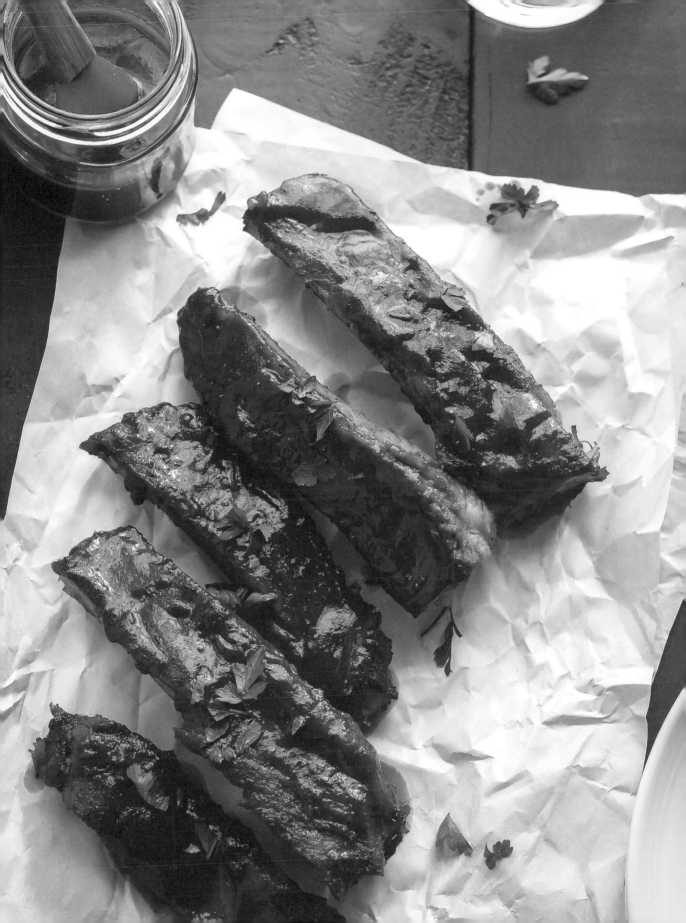

7 Transfer the pork to a chopping board. Pour the sauce through a sieve and into a small saucepan. Rapidly boil over medium–high heat until it reduces to a moderately thick sauce (this will take 10–15 minutes).

8 Increase the oven temperature to 425°F. Line a baking sheet with parchment paper.

9 Gently cut the ribs into single portions. Place on the prepared baking sheet and coat each rib with sauce (use about half of the sauce). Bake for another 10–15 minutes, basting a couple of times with the remaining sauce. Cook until the pork is delightfully sticky! Or baste the ribs and cook on the barbecue for a few minutes on each side.

10 Serve hot with your favorite low-FODMAP sides.

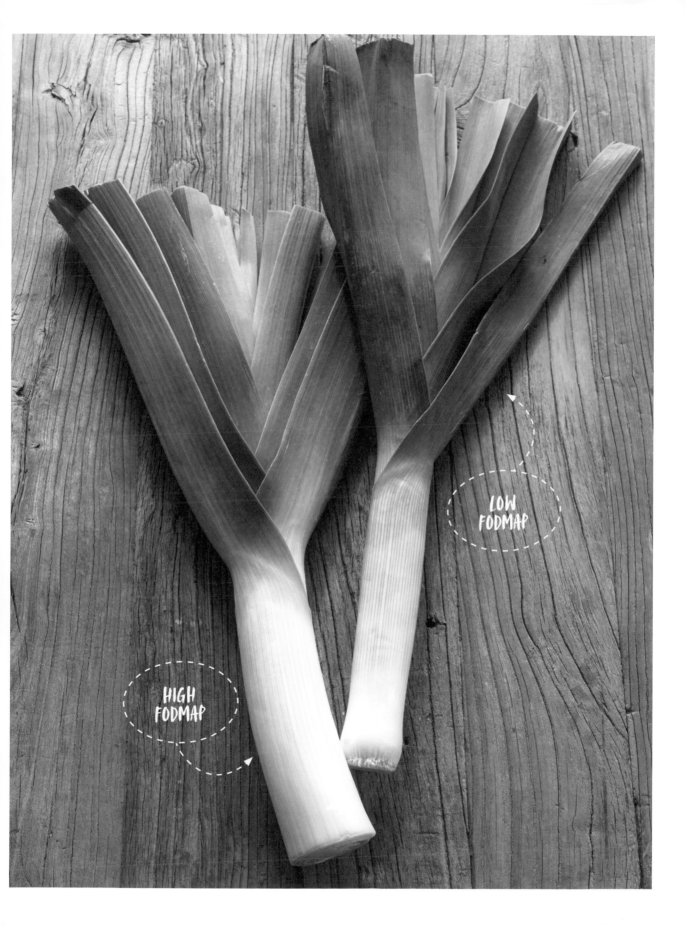

LOW
FODMAP

HIGH
FODMAP

Lemongrass & Cilantro Pork Meatballs with Stir-Fried Veggies

PREP TIME: 20 minutes **COOK TIME**: 20 minutes
SERVES: 4

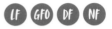

1¼ cups long-grain white rice or basmati rice

MEATBALLS

1 pound (450g) lean ground pork

3½ tablespoons chopped fresh cilantro

2 tablespoons chopped fresh lemongrass

¼ teaspoon crushed red pepper* (optional)

2 tablespoons brown sugar

½ cup gluten-free breadcrumbs*

1 tablespoon garlic-infused oil*

1 large egg, lightly beaten

A few grinds of salt and pepper

Drizzle of neutral oil (e.g. canola, grapeseed, safflower, sunflower)

STIR-FRIED VEGGIES

1 tablespoon sesame oil

Thumb-sized piece of fresh ginger, cut into matchsticks

2 large (8½oz/240g) carrots, peeled and cut into matchsticks

¼ cup finely sliced scallions (green leaves only)

4 cups (12oz/340g) sliced bok choy

3 tablespoons soy sauce (GF if needed)

1 tablespoon water

TIPS
*Check buying tips (see pages 25–26).

These low-FODMAP lemongrass and cilantro pork meatballs are an easy Asian-inspired dish!

1 In a large saucepan, cook the rice according to package instructions.

2 To make the meatballs, place the ground pork, cilantro, lemongrass, crushed red pepper (if using), brown sugar, breadcrumbs, garlic-infused oil, and egg in a large bowl. Season with salt and pepper. Mix well using your hands. Roll into bite-sized balls (should make about six per serving).

3 Heat the neutral oil in a large frying pan or wok over medium heat. When hot, fry the meatballs until they are golden brown on all sides and cooked through. Remove from the pan and keep warm.

4 Place the same frying pan over high heat. Add the sesame oil, ginger, carrot, and scallions. Cook until fragrant (1–2 minutes). Add the bok choy, soy sauce, and water. Stir-fry for 1–2 minutes and serve immediately.

5 Serve the rice in bowls and top with stir-fried veggies and pork meatballs.

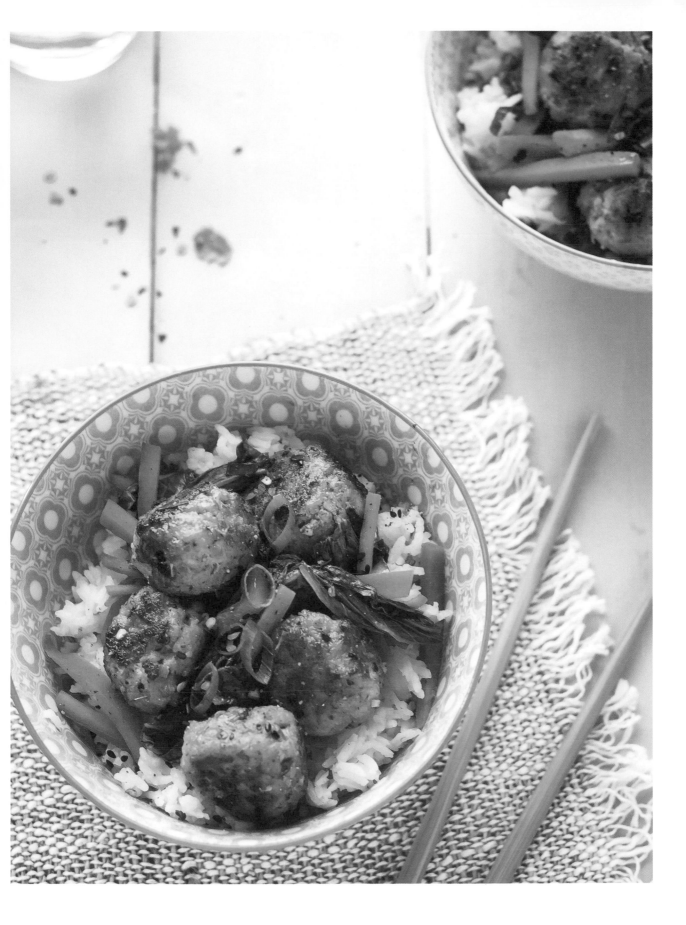

Basil Pesto Pasta

PREP TIME: 10 minutes **COOK TIME:** 10 minutes
SERVES: 4

LF **GF** **DFO** **EF** **NF** **SF**

9 ounces (260g) gluten-free penne pasta*

Drizzle of olive oil

½ pound (225g) lean bacon,* rind removed and diced

3 cups (8½oz/240g) cubed eggplant

A few grinds of salt and pepper, to taste

3 cups (3oz/90g) roughly chopped baby spinach

¼ cup thinly sliced scallions (green leaves only)

3 tablespoons toasted pumpkin seeds

3 tablespoons Easy Basil Pesto (see recipe on page 215)

2 tablespoons dairy-free spread or butter

2 tablespoons roughly chopped flat-leaf parsley

Parmesan or Cheddar,* thinly sliced (optional)

My homemade basil pesto is a quick and easy way to whip up a last-minute pasta dish. Keep a jar of it handy in the fridge for this midweek meal.

1 Cook the pasta according to package instructions.

2 Heat the olive oil in a large frying pan over medium heat. Fry the bacon until crispy.

3 While the bacon cooks, place the eggplant on a baking sheet, toss with a drizzle of olive oil, and season with salt and pepper. Grill until golden brown and soft, turning once (this will take about 8 minutes).

4 Add the grilled eggplant, spinach, scallions, and pumpkin seeds to the cooked bacon and cook for 1–2 minutes.

5 Drain the pasta and toss with the bacon and veggies, pesto, and dairy-free spread or butter.

6 Serve in bowls and top with parsley and slices of cheese, if using. Season with salt and pepper.

TIPS
*Check buying tips (see pages 25–26).

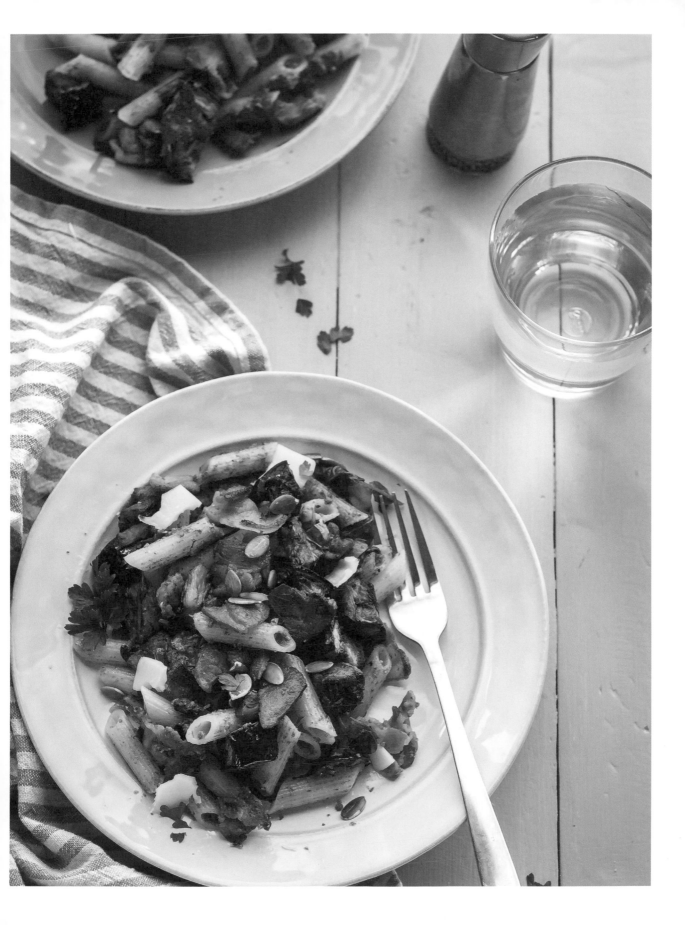

Pumpkin & Sage Pasta with Crispy Bacon

PREP TIME: 15 minutes **COOK TIME:** 30 minutes
SERVES: 4

LF GF DFO EF NF SF

2 cups (8½oz/240g) peeled and diced kabocha squash/Japanese pumpkin

2 large (8½oz/240g) carrots, peeled and cubed

1 tablespoon olive oil

½ pound (225g) lean bacon,* rind removed and cut into small pieces

¾ cup (2oz/60g) finely chopped leeks (green leaves only)

1 tablespoon garlic-infused oil*

3 tablespoons chopped fresh sage

A few grinds of salt and pepper

2 cups (500ml) low-FODMAP chicken or vegetable stock* (GF if needed)

10 ounces (280g) gluten-free spaghetti*

4 cups (4oz/120g) roughly chopped baby spinach

2 tablespoons grated Parmesan, mozzarella, or vegan cheese* (optional)

This creamy pumpkin sauce goes perfectly with bacon and pasta to create a delicious low-FODMAP meal. Make sure you use fresh sage to give this dish lots of flavor.

1 Place the pumpkin and carrot in a microwave-proof bowl with 2 tablespoons of water and cook on high for 2–3 minutes.

2 Heat the olive oil in a large frying pan over medium–high heat. Add the bacon and cook until crispy. Set aside and keep warm.

3 Add the precooked carrot and pumpkin, leeks, garlic-infused oil, and 2 tablespoons of the sage to the frying pan. Season with salt and pepper and cook for 5 minutes, stirring occasionally. Add the stock, bring to a boil, then reduce the heat and simmer until the carrot is soft and the liquid has reduced by almost half (about 10 minutes). Remove from the heat and leave to cool for 5 minutes.

4 Cook the pasta according to package instructions. Once cooked, drain and reserve 1 cup of the pasta water.

5 Place the cooled pumpkin and carrot mixture in a blender and blend until smooth. (Alternatively, you could do this in a bowl using an immersion blender.) Return the puree to the large frying pan and thin it with ¼ cup of pasta water (add a little more water as needed). Toss the pasta in the sauce and add the spinach.

6 Serve topped with bacon and sprinkled with cheese (if desired) and the remaining chopped sage.

TIPS
*Check buying tips (see pages 25–26).

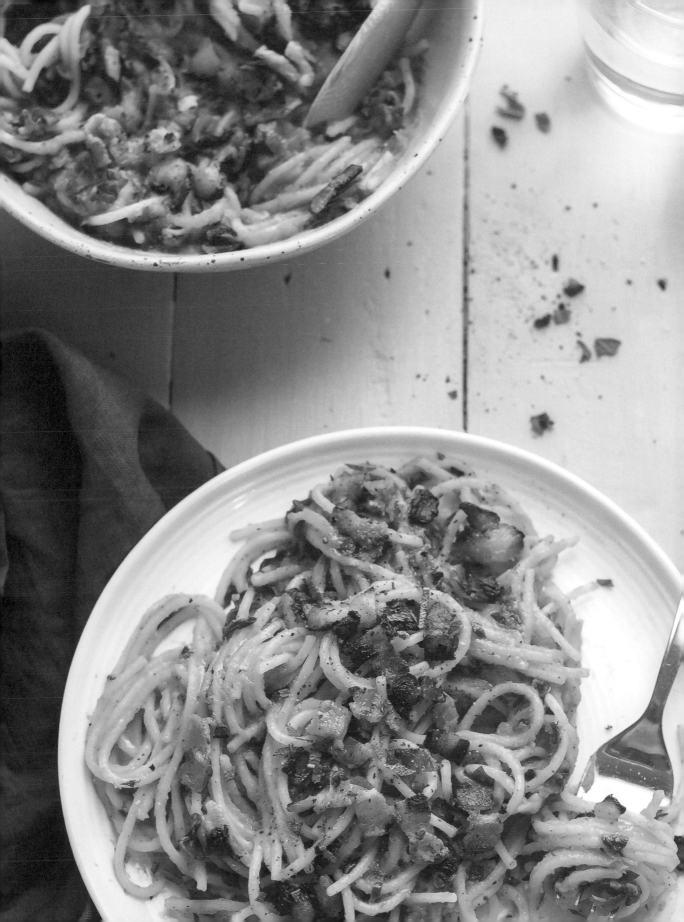

Minestrone Soup

PREP TIME: 20 minutes COOK TIME: 30 minutes
SERVES: 4

(LF) (GF) (DFO) (EF) (NF) (SF)

1 tablespoon garlic-infused oil*

2 large (8½oz/240g) carrots, peeled and diced

2 slices (2oz/65g) lean bacon,* rind removed and diced

1 small (5½oz/160g) potato, peeled and diced

1 stick (1½oz/50g) celery, sliced

1 cup (2½oz/80g) finely chopped leeks (green leaves only)

Drizzle of olive oil

1 cup (6oz/170g) canned chickpeas (measure after draining and rinsing)

1 (15oz/400g) can plain crushed/ chopped tomatoes

2 cups (500ml) low-FODMAP chicken or vegetable stock* (GF if needed)

1¼ cups (310ml) boiling water

1½ cups (5½oz/165g) diced zucchini

2 cups (2oz/60g) roughly chopped spinach

1 cup (2½oz/75g) gluten-free pasta spirals or shells*

½ cup lightly packed fresh basil

A few grinds of salt and pepper, to taste

Drizzle of garlic-infused oil,* to serve

Grated Parmesan or vegan cheese,* to serve (optional)

This low-FODMAP soup is kid approved and bowl-licking good. To make this dish vegetarian, just leave out the bacon.

1 Heat the garlic-infused oil in a large saucepan over medium heat. Add the carrot, bacon, potato, celery, and leeks. Sauté gently for 15–20 minutes, until the ingredients start to soften. Add a drizzle of olive oil and turn down the heat if needed (the vegetables should be soft but not too brown).

2 While the veggies cook, drain and rinse the chickpeas.

3 Add the tomatoes, stock, hot water, zucchini, spinach, and chickpeas to the pan. Bring to a boil and simmer over medium–low heat for 10 minutes.

4 Measure out the pasta and roughly chop the basil (leaves and stalks). Reserve a few small basil leaves for the garnish.

5 Add the pasta and basil to the soup. Cook the pasta in the soup according to package instructions, or until the pasta is cooked (if you are using the soup for lunches, undercook the pasta by 1–2 minutes to prevent it from turning mushy). If the soup is too thick, add a little water.

6 Season with salt and pepper. Garnish with reserved basil leaves and add a drizzle of garlic-infused oil and a sprinkle of Parmesan or vegan cheese, if desired.

TIPS
*Check buying tips (see pages 25–26).

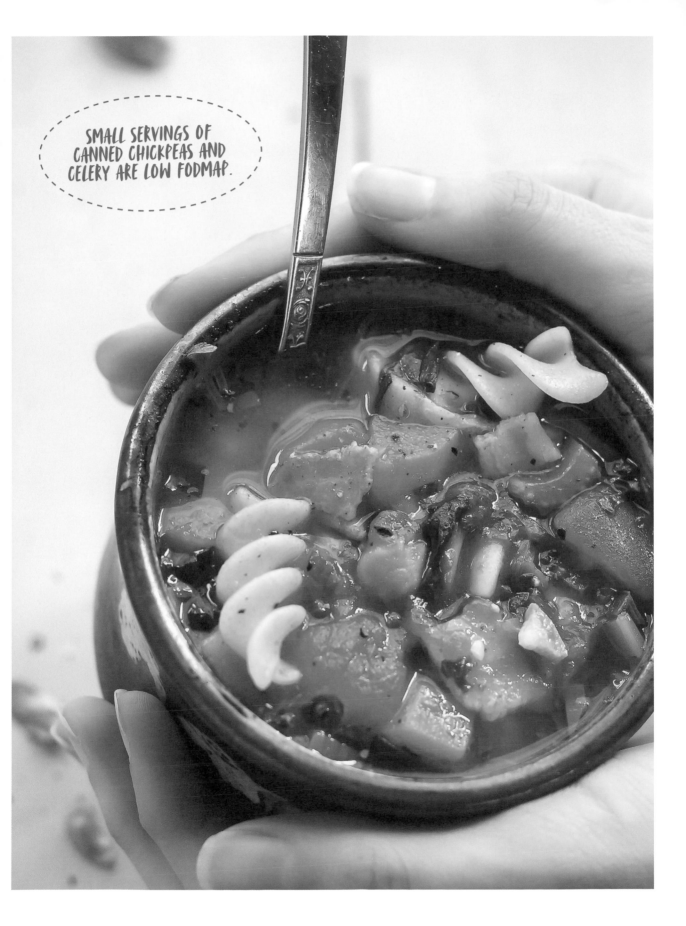

SMALL SERVINGS OF CANNED CHICKPEAS AND CELERY ARE LOW FODMAP.

Jamaican Pulled Pork with Salsa

PREP TIME: 15 minutes **COOK TIME:** 10 hours
SERVES: 6

LF GF DF EF NF SF

1¼ pounds (600g) pork shoulder roast,
  skin removed and fat trimmed
3 teaspoons paprika
2 teaspoons dried thyme
1 teaspoon allspice
1 teaspoon ground cinnamon
1 teaspoon dried chives
Pinch of crushed red pepper* (optional)
2 tablespoons brown sugar
3 tablespoons tomato paste
2 teaspoons crushed ginger*
2 cups (500ml) low-FODMAP chicken
  stock* (GF if needed)
1 cup (2½oz/80g) finely chopped leeks
  (green leaves only)
3 large (12½oz/360g) carrots, peeled
  and diced
1¾ cups long-grain white rice or
  basmati rice
A few grinds of salt and pepper, to taste
2 teaspoons garlic-infused oil*
2 teaspoons corn starch (GF if needed)

PINEAPPLE SALSA

1 red bell pepper, seeded and diced
1 (16oz/440g) can pineapple chunks in
  syrup,* drained, rinsed, and diced
¼ cup finely sliced scallions (green
  leaves only)
3 tablespoons finely chopped fresh
  cilantro

TIPS

*Check buying tips (see pages
25–26).

This slow-cooked, Jamaican-inspired pulled pork has yummy hints of cinnamon, paprika, and allspice, as well as a little heat. It's delicious with a fresh pineapple salsa and plain rice. Make at least six servings, as the leftovers are fantastic for sandwiches.

1 Place the pork in the slow cooker. Mix together the paprika, thyme, allspice, cinnamon, chives, crushed red pepper (if using), brown sugar, and tomato paste, then rub on the pork. Add the ginger, chicken stock, leeks, and carrot to the slow cooker. Cook for 10 hours on low or 5–6 hours on high.

2 Thirty minutes before you are ready to eat, cook the rice according to package instructions.

3 Make the salsa by placing all ingredients in a bowl and mixing well.

4 In the slow cooker, shred the pork using two forks, season with salt and pepper, then drizzle with garlic-infused oil. Remove the carrot and pork (leave the juices behind) and place on a baking sheet. Place under the oven grill and cook on high for 5–8 minutes, until golden and slightly crispy (don't leave it unattended as it can burn quickly).

5 Pour the pork juices into a small saucepan. Dissolve the corn starch in 2 tablespoons of cold water and mix. Simmer the gravy over medium heat for 3–4 minutes, until it has reached your desired thickness.

6 Serve the pulled pork with the rice, pineapple salsa, and gravy.

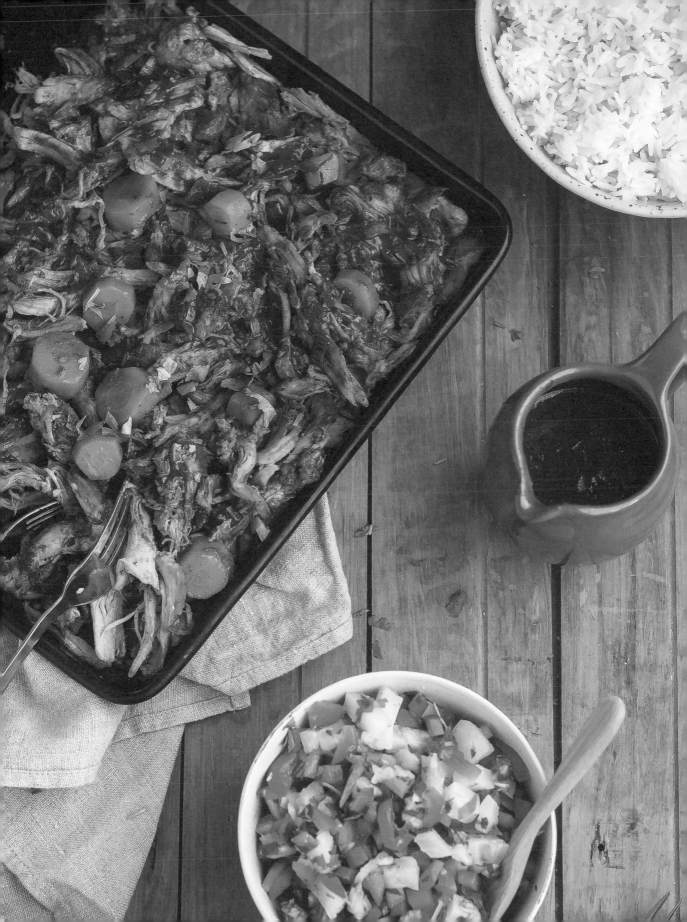

Pork Chops with Herb Mustard Sauce & Creamy Mash

PREP TIME: 10 minutes **COOK TIME**: 30 minutes
SERVES: 4

LF **GF** **DFO** **EF** **NF** **SF**

1¾ pounds (800g) potatoes, peeled
   and chopped
4 pork loin chops
Drizzle of neutral oil (e.g. canola,
   grapeseed, safflower, sunflower)
A few grinds of salt and pepper
1½ cups (6oz/180g) chopped green
   beans (cut into bite-sized pieces)
2 cups (6oz/180g) broccoli florets
2 tablespoons dairy-free spread or
   butter
¼ cup (60ml) low-FODMAP milk*
½ teaspoon salt

HERB MUSTARD SAUCE

4 tablespoons dairy-free spread or
   butter
1½ tablespoons Dijon mustard*
½ tablespoons pure maple syrup
½ teaspoon dried sage
4 tablespoons finely chopped fresh
   parsley
1 teaspoon corn starch (GF if needed)

These herb mustard pork chops are my mom's favorite low-FODMAP meal. I created a low-FODMAP twist on a honey mustard sauce by using pure maple syrup instead of honey.

1 Cook the potatoes in a large saucepan of boiling water until tender (about 15–20 minutes).

2 While the potatoes cook, make the herb mustard sauce and pan-fry the pork.

3 Place a small saucepan over medium–low heat and add the dairy-free spread or butter, mustard, maple syrup, sage, and parsley. Stir until combined. Dissolve the corn starch in warm water to form a paste before adding it to the sauce. Stir well and then leave over low heat, stirring occasionally, until thickened. Set aside.

4 Preheat a large frying pan over medium–high heat. As it heats, dry the pork chops with a paper towel then rub with a drizzle of neutral oil, salt, and pepper. Fry the pork chops over medium–high heat for 5 minutes on each side. Check the thickest piece of pork to make sure it is cooked right through (it should be white, not pink, right through). Rest them for 5 minutes.

5 While the pork rests, blanch the green beans and broccoli in boiling water for 2–3 minutes, until they are tender and bright green.

6 Drain the potatoes. Add the dairy-free spread or butter, milk, and salt. Mash until smooth.

7 Serve the pork with the herb mustard sauce, mashed potatoes, and veggies.

TIPS
*Check buying tips (see pages 26–27).

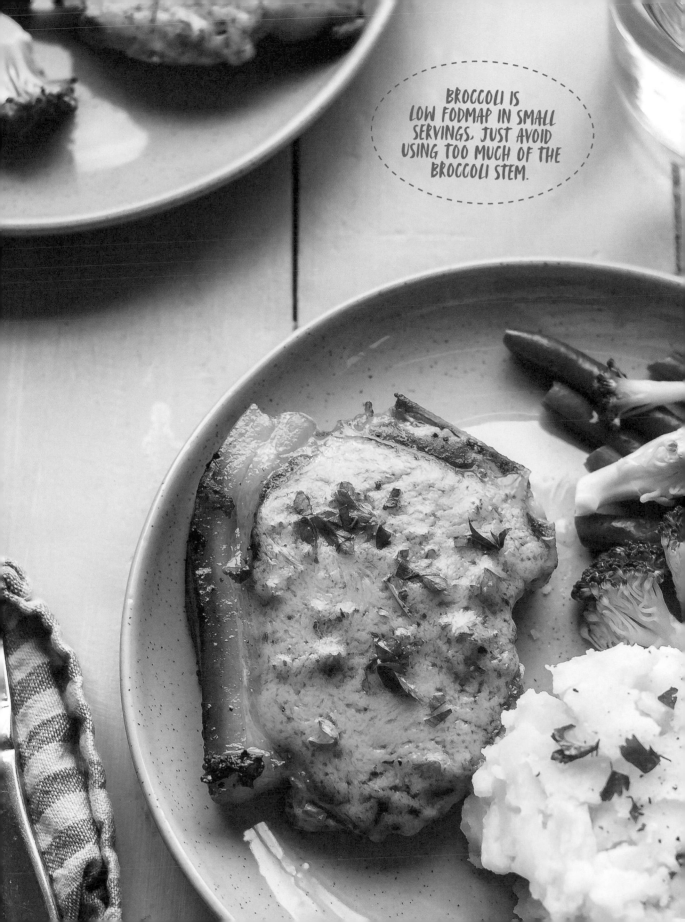

BROCCOLI IS LOW FODMAP IN SMALL SERVINGS. JUST AVOID USING TOO MUCH OF THE BROCCOLI STEM.

Fish with Pineapple Basil Salsa & Crunchy Wedges

PREP TIME: 15 minutes **COOK TIME:** 40 minutes
SERVES: 4

LF GF DFO EF NF SF

PAPRIKA WEDGES

1¼ pounds (600g) potatoes, peeled
Drizzle of neutral oil (e.g. canola,
    grapeseed, safflower, sunflower)
½ teaspoon paprika
A few grinds of salt and pepper

PINEAPPLE BASIL SALSA

2 medium tomatoes, diced
1 red bell pepper, seeded and diced
Handful of fresh basil, finely sliced
¼ cup finely chopped scallions (green
    leaves only)
1 (16oz/440g) can pineapple chunks in
    syrup,* drained, rinsed, and diced
3 teaspoons lemon juice
½ teaspoon white sugar
A few grinds of salt and pepper, to
    taste

CUMIN-SPICED FISH

4 tablespoons gluten-free all-purpose
    flour*
½ teaspoon ground cumin
1 pound (450g) mild white-fleshed fish
    fillets (such as cod or sea robin)
2 tablespoons dairy-free spread or
    butter, for cooking
4 cups shredded lettuce (e.g. butter,
    iceberg, red leaf), to serve

I love combining the tangy flavors of pineapple and basil salsa with cumin-spiced fish! This recipe creates a delicious, light meal. When you're shopping for firm, white fish, sea robin (also known as gurnard) is a great sustainable option.

1 Preheat oven to 400°F. Line a baking sheet with parchment paper.

2 Cut the potatoes into wedges, pat dry with a paper towel, and place on the prepared baking sheet. Drizzle with oil, sprinkle with paprika, and season with salt and pepper. Cook in the oven until golden (30–40 minutes). Turn once during cooking.

3 Make the salsa by placing all the ingredients in a bowl. Mix well and set aside.

4 To prepare the fish, place the flour, cumin, and a few grinds of salt and pepper in a large bowl. Mix well. Coat each side of the fish fillets with the flour mixture.

5 Just as the wedges finish cooking, place a large frying pan over medium heat. Heat the dairy-free spread or butter in the pan, then fry each side of the fish for 2–3 minutes, until cooked through.

6 Serve the fish with the salsa, lettuce, and homemade wedges.

TIPS
*Check buying tips (see page 25).

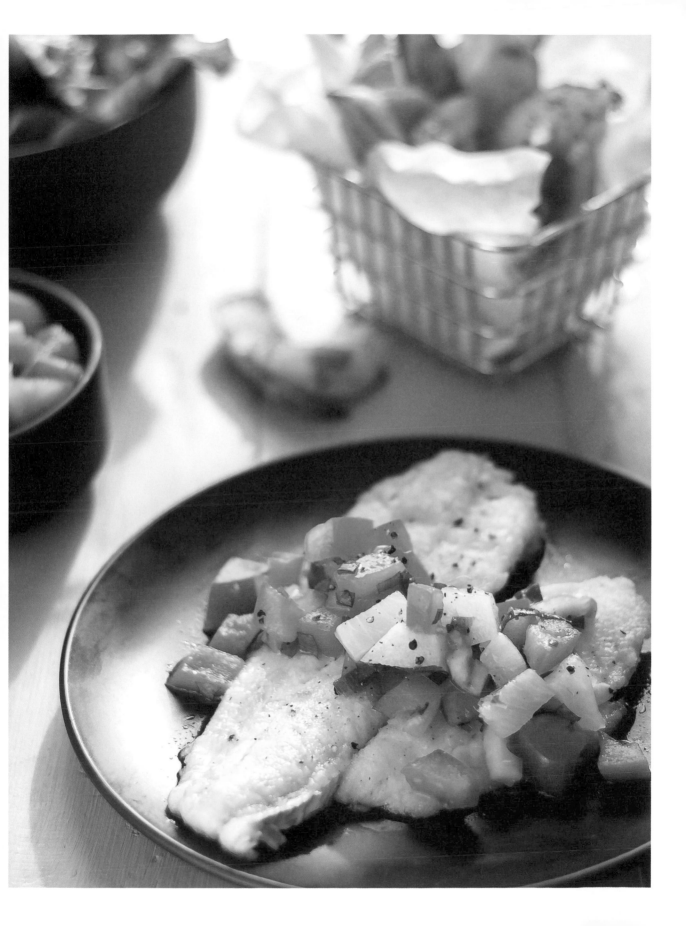

Mediterranean Pan-Fried Fish

PREP TIME: 10 minutes **COOK TIME:** 25 minutes
SERVES: 4

(LF) (GF) (DFO) (EF) (NF) (SF)

1¼ cups long-grain white rice or
   basmati rice
2 cups (5½oz/160g) thinly sliced then
   quartered eggplant
Drizzle of neutral oil (e.g. canola,
   grapeseed, safflower, sunflower)
A few grinds of salt and pepper
1¾ cups (8½oz/240g) sliced zucchini
   (cut into sticks)
3 cups (9oz/255g) chopped bok choy
   (stems and leaves separated)
3 tablespoons dairy-free spread or
   butter
½ cup (1oz/40g) thinly sliced leeks
   (green leaves only)
14 ounces (400g) mild white-fleshed
   fish fillets (such as snapper)
16 cherry tomatoes
3 teaspoons lemon zest
2 tablespoons lemon juice, or to taste
2 tablespoons chopped fresh parsley

I love the freshness and simplicity of Mediterranean food. The cherry tomatoes create delicious, juicy bursts, and I adore how the lemon zest gives the dish a light and refreshing twist.

1 Cook the rice according to package instructions.

2 Place the eggplant on a baking sheet, drizzle with oil, and season with salt and pepper. Grill in the oven under high heat for 4 minutes on each side, until soft and golden.

3 Heat a drizzle of oil in a medium frying pan over medium heat. Stir-fry the zucchini and bok choy stems for 8–10 minutes, until golden brown. Season with salt and pepper. Then add the bok choy leaves and stir-fry for 1–2 minutes.

4 Heat the dairy-free spread or butter in a large frying pan over medium heat. Add the leeks and fry for 1 minute, stirring frequently. Add the fish and cherry tomatoes. Fry the fish for 2–3 minutes on each side. Add 2 teaspoons of the lemon zest to the pan, squeeze over 1 teaspoon of the lemon juice, and season with salt and pepper. Add the veggies from the baking sheet and gently mix together.

5 Serve the fish and veggies with the rice. Sprinkle with parsley and the remaining lemon zest. Squeeze over more lemon juice as needed.

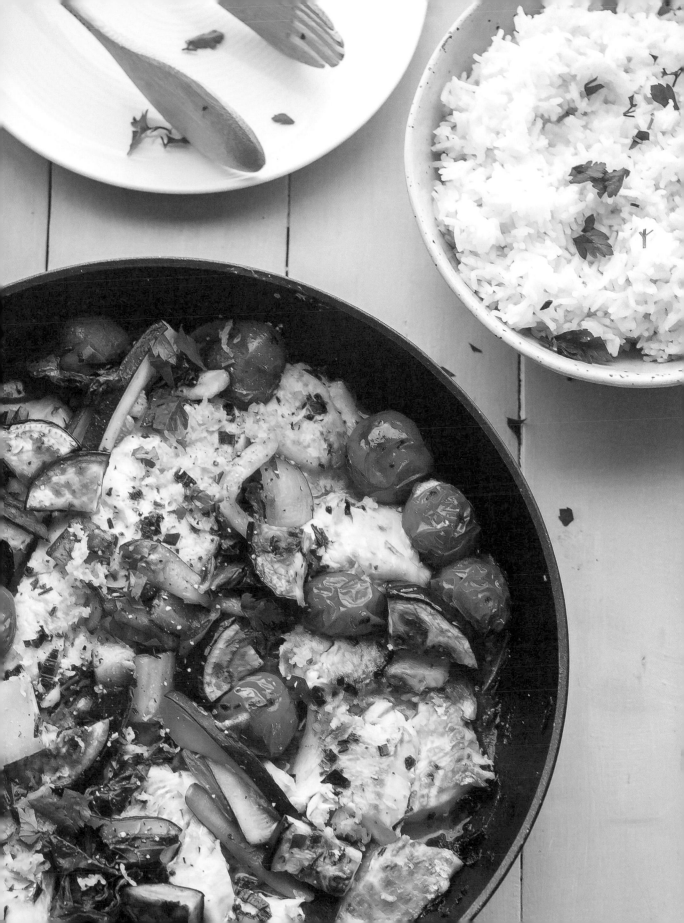

Sweet & Sticky Salmon Skewers

PREP TIME: 15 minutes + marinating time **COOK TIME**: 10 minutes
SERVES: 4

(LF) (GFO) (DF) (EF) (NF)

1 pound (450g) boneless, skinless
   fresh salmon fillets
2 teaspoons garlic-infused oil*
1½ teaspoons crushed ginger*
1½ tablespoons pure maple syrup
Zest and juice of 1 large lime
2 tablespoons soy sauce (GF if
   needed)
1 tablespoon sesame seeds

This maple soy marinade creates beautifully sweet and sticky salmon skewers. Cook these on the barbecue or under the oven grill for a tasty low-FODMAP salmon dish.

1 Soak four wooden skewers in a bowl of water for 10–15 minutes (this will help prevent burning).

2 Cut the salmon into 1-inch cubes. In a bowl, mix together the oil, ginger, maple syrup, lime zest and juice, and soy sauce. Place the salmon in the marinade and stir to coat. Marinate for 10 minutes.

3 Slide the salmon pieces onto the skewers. Place on a lightly oiled baking sheet and grill for 8–10 minutes, until cooked through. Turn three times during cooking (every couple of minutes), each time basting with more marinade. Alternatively, cook on the barbecue, basting the skewers each time you turn them.

4 While the salmon cooks, toast the sesame seeds in a dry pan over medium–high heat for 1–2 minutes, until golden.

5 Garnish each salmon skewer with a sprinkle of toasted sesame seeds. Serve with a side of rice and stir-fried veggies (bok choy and bell pepper are good), or with Caramelized Beet, Pumpkin & Feta Salad (see recipe on page 74).

TIPS
*Check buying tips (see page 25).

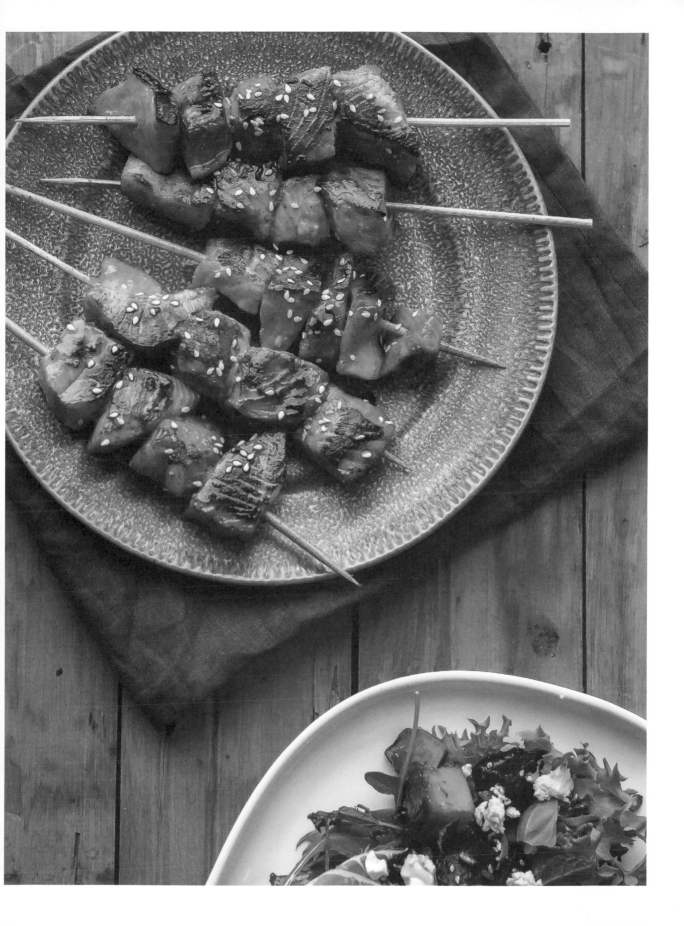

20-Minute Vegan Pasta

PREP TIME: 5 minutes **COOK TIME**: 15 minutes
SERVES: 4

(LF) (GF) (DF) (EF) (NF) (SF)

1 tablespoon garlic-infused oil*

1 cup (2½oz/80g) finely chopped leeks
   (green leaves only)

1 (15oz/400g) can plain crushed/
   chopped tomatoes

1½ tablespoons tomato paste

1½ cups (375ml) low-FODMAP
   vegetable stock* (GF if needed)

4 cups (4oz/120g) finely chopped
   spinach

1 teaspoon white sugar

1 dried bay leaf

A few grinds of salt and pepper

1 teaspoon corn starch (GF if needed)

1 cup (6oz/170g) canned chickpeas
   (measure after draining and rinsing)

4 tablespoons sunflower seeds

½ pound (225g) gluten-free pasta*

½ cup (2oz/55g) grated vegan
   cheese* or mozzarella

Who doesn't love a 20-minute meal?! My roommates like to describe this low-FODMAP vegan pasta dish as one that won't scare away the meat-eaters. Personally, I love it because it's quick and doesn't need too many ingredients.

1 Bring a large saucepan of water to a boil (you will use this for the pasta).

2 Heat the oil in a medium saucepan over medium heat. Add the leeks and fry for 2–3 minutes, until fragrant. Add the tomatoes, tomato paste, stock, spinach, sugar, and bay leaf and season with salt and pepper. Simmer for 15 minutes, stirring occasionally.

3 Dissolve the corn starch in a small amount of cold water and mix it in with the sauce along with the chickpeas. Allow to thicken for 1–2 minutes, then remove the bay leaf.

4 While the sauce simmers, roughly chop the sunflower seeds and toast them in a small frying pan (no oil) over medium–low heat for 2–3 minutes, until golden brown. Tip onto a plate and set aside.

5 Cook the pasta according to package instructions, then drain.

6 Toss the sauce in the pasta, top with vegan cheese or mozzarella, and garnish with sunflower seeds.

TIPS
*Check buying tips (see pages 25–26).

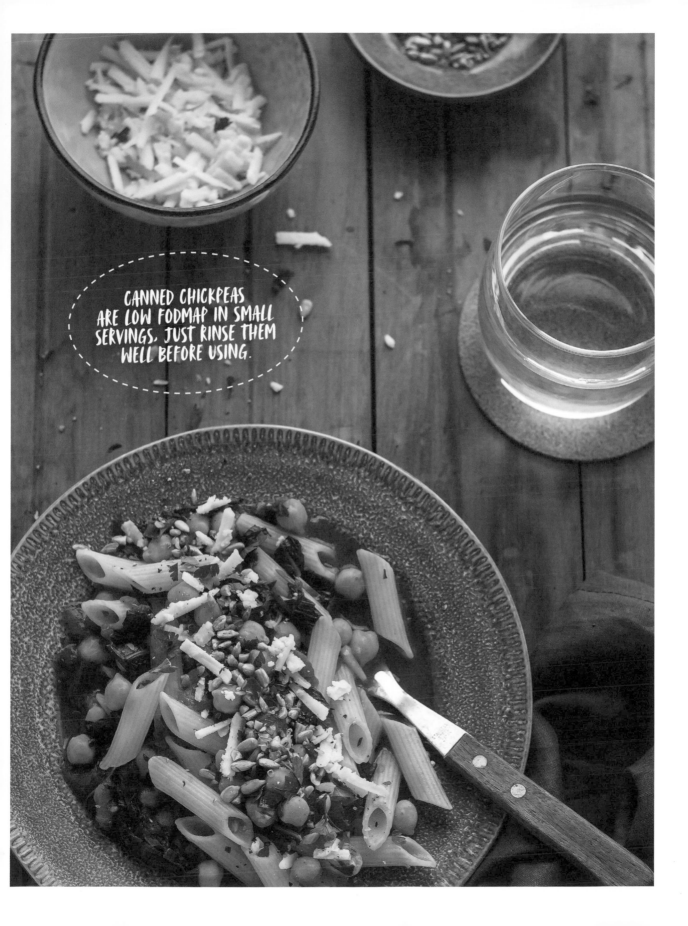

CANNED CHICKPEAS ARE LOW FODMAP IN SMALL SERVINGS, JUST RINSE THEM WELL BEFORE USING.

Pumpkin & Carrot Risotto

PREP TIME: 15 minutes COOK TIME: 45 minutes
SERVES: 4

LF GF DFO EF NF SFO

2 cups (8½oz/240g) peeled and diced kabocha squash/Japanese pumpkin

2 large (8½oz/240g) carrots, peeled and cut into small pieces

1 tablespoon olive oil

A few grinds of salt and pepper

½ cup (1oz/40g) finely chopped leeks (green leaves only)

1 tablespoon garlic-infused oil*

1 tablespoon dairy-free spread or butter

1½ cups arborio rice

4 cups low-FODMAP chicken or vegetable stock* (GF if needed), heated

4 cups (4oz/120g) finely chopped spinach

2½ tablespoons lemon juice

2 teaspoons lemon zest

2 ounces (50g) Parmesan or vegan cheese,* grated (optional)

2 tablespoons chopped fresh cilantro or parsley

This creamy pumpkin and carrot risotto combines fresh lemon flavors with sweet roasted veggies and is a favorite comfort dish of mine. This dish is great on its own or paired with pan-fried, white-fleshed fish.

1 Preheat oven to 400°F. Place the pumpkin and carrots in a roasting pan, drizzle with olive oil, and season with salt and pepper. Bake for 20–25 minutes (until soft and slightly golden). Toss a couple of times during cooking.

2 While the veggies are cooking, make the risotto. Heat a large saucepan over medium heat. Add the leeks, oil, and dairy-free spread or butter to the pan and fry for 2 minutes, until fragrant. Add the rice, stirring it in the mixture for about 1 minute.

3 Add ½ cup of hot stock, stirring every now and then until the liquid has been absorbed. Continue adding and stirring in the stock, a ½ cup at a time, waiting until it has been absorbed before adding the next ½ cup. Turn down the heat to medium–low if needed (if the rice is cooking too quickly and starting to stick to the bottom of the pan). Once the rice has absorbed about three-quarters of the stock (this should take about 20 minutes), check to see if the rice is tender. If it isn't, add more stock and continue cooking for another few minutes.

4 While the rice finishes cooking, stir in the spinach, lemon juice, and lemon zest. Season with salt and pepper. Stir in the roasted veggies and cheese, if using.

5 Serve the risotto in bowls and garnish with fresh cilantro or parsley.

TIPS
*Check buying tips (see pages 25–26).

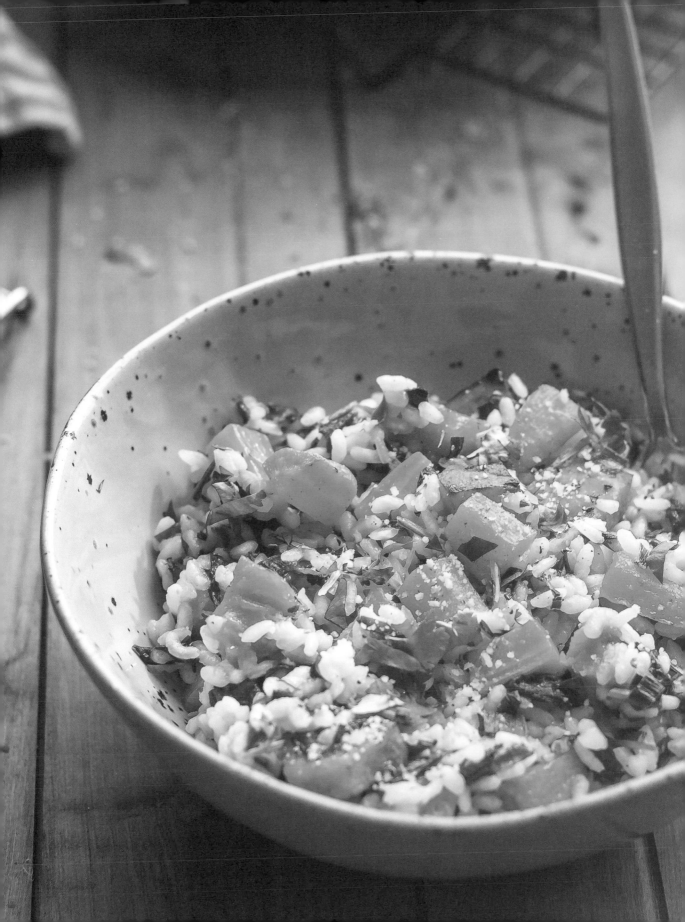

Hummus Buddha Bowl

PREP TIME: 10 minutes **COOK TIME:** 30 minutes
SERVES: 4

(LF) (GF) (DF) (EF) (NF) (SF)

CUMIN-ROASTED CARROTS

2 large (8½oz/240g) carrots, peeled
Drizzle of olive oil
1 teaspoon ground cumin
A few grinds of salt and pepper

LEMON TAHINI DRESSING

1 tablespoon tahini
1 tablespoon lemon juice
1 tablespoon olive oil
½ tablespoon pure maple syrup

BUDDHA BOWL

4 tablespoons pumpkin seeds
2 cups cooked brown rice
3 cups (3oz/90g) roughly chopped
   baby spinach
20 cherry tomatoes, halved
½ cup (1½oz/45g) shredded red
   cabbage (optional)
8 tablespoons Traditional Hummus
   (see recipe on page 210;
   2 tablespoons per serving)
1 mild green chile, thinly sliced
   (optional)

Buddha bowls are a delicious way to create nutrient-packed meals. They are also ideal for using leftover low-FODMAP vegetables.

1 Preheat oven to 350°F. Slice the carrots into thick sticks. Place on a baking sheet and toss with olive oil, cumin, and salt and pepper. Roast for 25 minutes, until soft and golden.

2 Make the lemon tahini dressing by whisking together all the dressing ingredients in a small bowl or jar.

3 Toast the pumpkin seeds in a dry pan over medium heat for 1–2 minutes, until golden, then roughly chop.

4 Assemble by dividing the roasted carrots, cooked rice, baby spinach, cherry tomatoes, red cabbage, and hummus evenly among four bowls. Garnish with toasted pumpkin seeds and a few slices of green chile, if desired. Drizzle with lemon tahini dressing.

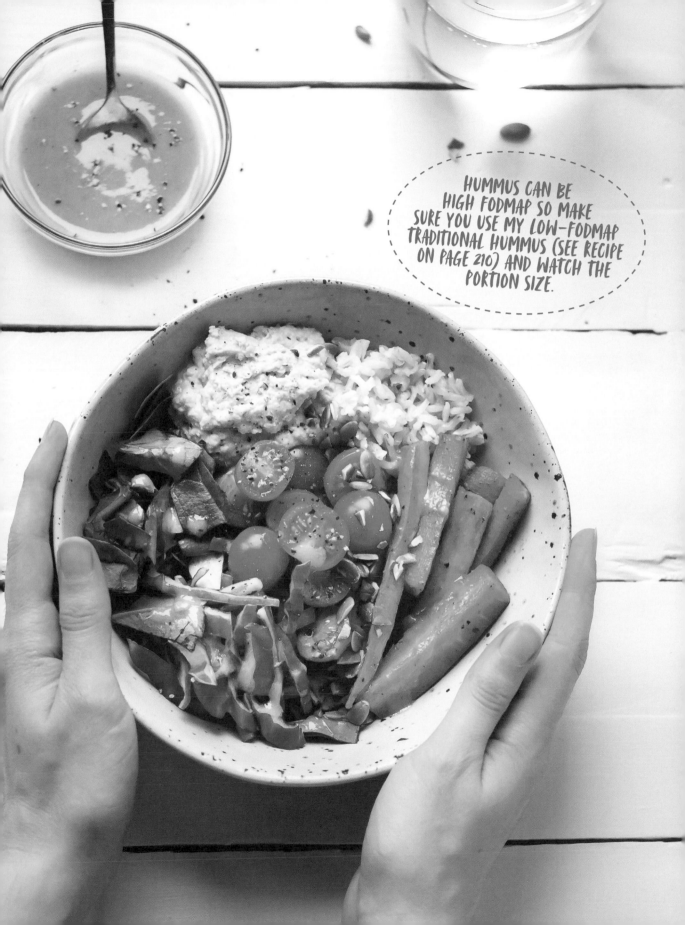

HUMMUS CAN BE HIGH FODMAP SO MAKE SURE YOU USE MY LOW-FODMAP TRADITIONAL HUMMUS (SEE RECIPE ON PAGE 210) AND WATCH THE PORTION SIZE.

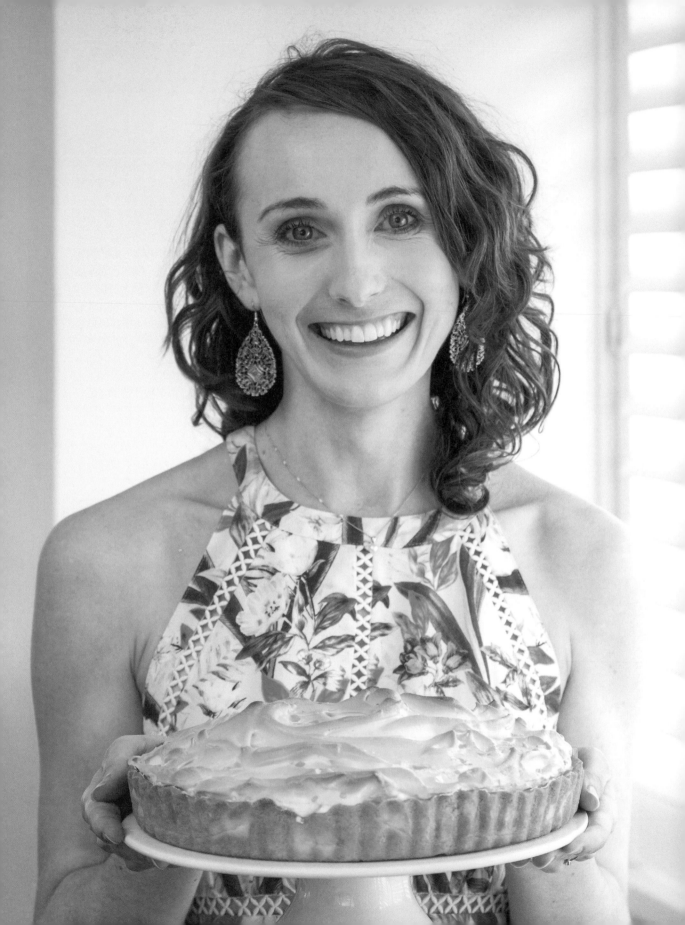

SWEET TREATS

Sometimes all you need in life
is a sweet treat, and I've got an
option for every occasion.

Dark Chocolate & Raspberry Muffins

PREP TIME: 10 minutes **COOK TIME**: 20 minutes
MAKES: 12 muffins

(LF) (GF) (DFO) (EFO) (NF) (SF)

2½ cups (350g) gluten-free self-rising
    flour*
6 tablespoons (100g) dairy-free spread
    or butter, chopped and softened
1 cup (210g) white sugar
1 cup (250ml) low-FODMAP milk*
2 large eggs, lightly beaten
1 teaspoon guar gum or xanthan gum
    (or 1 teaspoon chia seeds soaked in
    2 tablespoons hot water)
1 cup (4½oz/125g) fresh or frozen
    raspberries
½ cup (3oz/90g) chopped dark
    chocolate, cut into small pieces
Confectioners' sugar for dusting (GF if
    needed, optional)

These beautiful muffins are one of my favorite afternoon treats—you get the gorgeous tang of the raspberries coupled with the richness of the dark chocolate. They are also quick and easy to make!

1 Preheat oven to 375°F. Place the oven rack in the center of the oven. Grease a 12-hole muffin pan.

2 Place the flour in a large bowl. Rub the dairy-free spread or butter into the flour using your fingertips. Continue doing this until the mixture turns grainy with a few lumps and is well combined.

3 Add the sugar, milk, egg, gum (or chia seed mixture), raspberries, and chocolate to the flour mixture. Mix until it is just moistened.

4 Fill the muffin pan with the mixture (three-quarters of the way to the top).

5 Bake in the preheated oven for 15 minutes. Use a skewer to see if the centers are still gooey. If the skewer doesn't come out clean (don't worry about melted chocolate), then bake for another 2–5 minutes. The outsides of the muffins should be golden brown.

6 Leave the muffins in the pan for 5 minutes before transferring to a wire rack to cool slightly.

7 Serve warm and dust with confectioners' sugar, if desired.

TIPS

These muffins are best warm, so reheat them in the microwave for 20 seconds before serving. To make this recipe egg free, you can replace the eggs with a commercial egg replacer.

*Check buying tips (see pages 25–27).

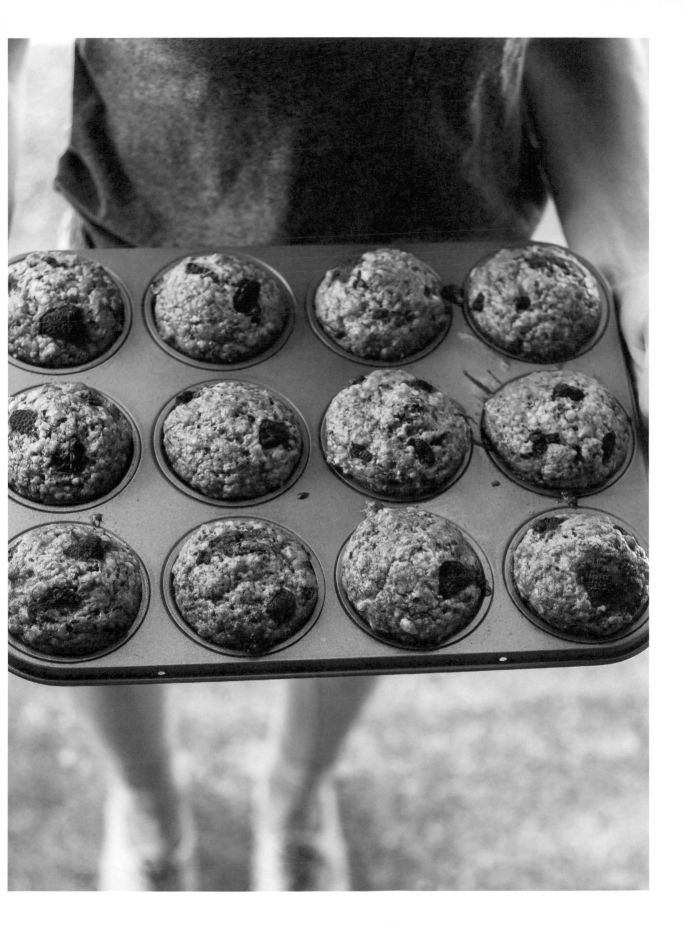

Birthday Banana Cake with Lemon Icing

PREP TIME: 15 minutes **COOK TIME:** 60 minutes + cooling time
SERVES: 16 (limit 1 slice per serving)

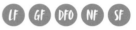

½ pound (2 sticks/250g) dairy-free spread or butter, cubed

1 cup (210g) white sugar

2 teaspoons vanilla essence

3 large eggs

2 cups (3–4 large) mashed firm banana (no brown spots)

2 teaspoons lemon juice

1 teaspoon chia seeds

2 tablespoons boiling water

½ cup (125ml) low-FODMAP milk*

2 teaspoons baking soda (GF if needed)

3 cups (420g) gluten-free all-purpose flour*

2 teaspoons baking powder (GF if needed)

LEMON ICING

5 tablespoons (80g) dairy-free spread or butter, softened

1½ cups (195g) confectioners' sugar (GF if needed)

1½ tablespoons lemon juice

1 tablespoon lemon zest

TIPS
*Check buying tips (see pages 25–27).

I made this gorgeous banana cake with lemon icing for my birthday. It has sweetness from the bananas and tanginess from the lemons, which makes it absolutely delicious!

1 Preheat oven to 350°F. Place the oven rack in the center of the oven. Grease and line a 10-inch round cake pan with parchment paper.

2 Slightly soften the dairy-free spread or butter (but don't melt it). Cream the dairy-free spread or butter and sugar together in a large bowl until fluffy. Beat in the vanilla essence and the eggs, adding one egg at a time.

3 Mix the banana and the lemon juice in the wet mixture. Soften the chia seeds in the boiling water until thickened. Then stir them in the wet mixture.

4 Heat the milk in the microwave for 20 seconds. Stir the baking soda into the milk. Fold in the wet mixture.

5 Sift the flour into a large bowl and stir through the baking powder. Combine the dry and wet mixtures. Mix gently until just combined.

6 Pour the cake batter into the prepared cake pan.

7 Bake in the preheated oven for 45–60 minutes, until the top is golden, the cake feels spongy to the touch, and a toothpick inserted in the middle comes out clean. Leave the cake to cool before icing.

8 To make the icing, place the dairy-free spread or butter, confectioners' sugar, lemon juice, and half of the lemon zest in a large bowl and beat until smooth and creamy. If the mixture isn't wet enough, add a small squeeze of lemon juice. Frost the cake and sprinkle with the remaining lemon zest.

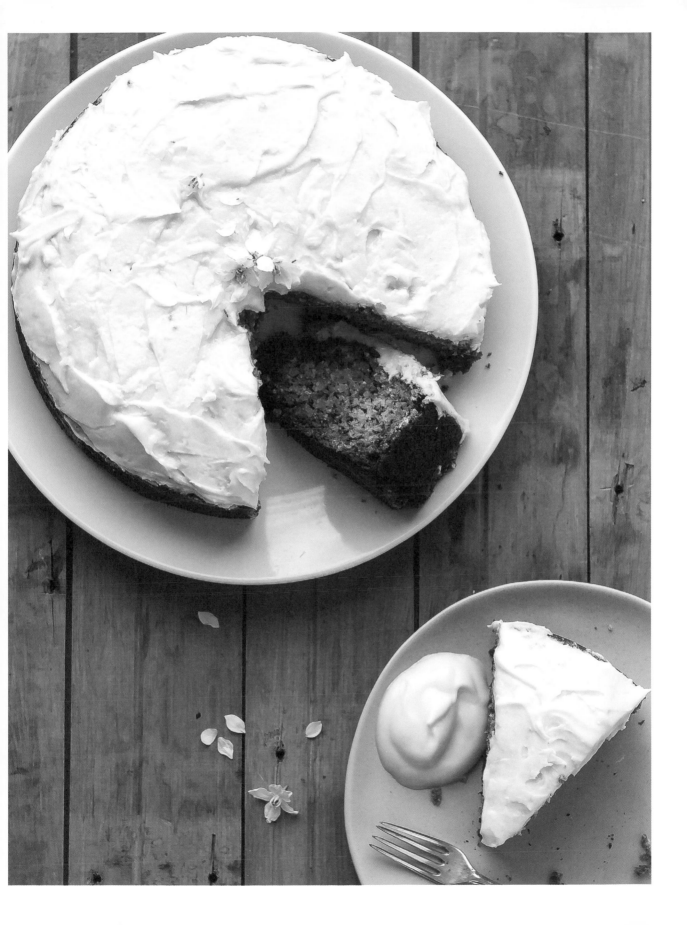

Blueberry Crumble Slice

PREP TIME: 35 minutes **COOK TIME**: 30 minutes
SERVES: 15 (limit 1 slice per serving)

(LF) (GF) (DFO) (NF) (SF)

BASE

¾ cup (155g) white sugar

3 cups (420g) gluten-free self-rising flour*

¼ teaspoon salt

½ teaspoon ground cinnamon

1 teaspoon guar gum or xanthan gum (optional)

½ pound (2 sticks/250g) dairy-free spread or butter, cubed and softened

1 large egg

FILLING

3 cups (15½oz/445g) fresh or frozen blueberries

3 teaspoons corn starch (GF if needed)

¼ cup (55g) white sugar

This slice is incredibly yummy. No one will be able to tell that it's low FODMAP, and gluten and dairy free! It's perfect as an afternoon treat or dessert, and goes well with low-FODMAP yogurt.

1 Preheat oven to 350°F. Place the oven rack in the center of the oven. Grease an 8-by-12-inch baking pan or line with parchment paper.

2 Place the sugar, flour, salt, and cinnamon in a medium bowl and mix together well. If you are using gum, add it to the dry ingredients. The gum will make the mixture less crumbly.

3 Place the dairy-free spread or butter in a bowl and soften slightly in the microwave (do not melt). Using a fork, mix the dairy-free spread (or butter) and egg into the dry ingredients until well combined. Then rub the mixture between your fingers until it turns into large, moist crumbs.

4 Firmly pat half of the mixture into the pan until it forms a smooth layer. Spread the blueberries evenly on top to cover the dough.

5 Mix together the corn starch and sugar, and sprinkle evenly over the blueberries. Crumble the remaining dough over the top.

6 Bake in the preheated oven for 30 minutes or until the top is slightly golden. Leave the slice to cool before cutting it into 15 pieces. Serve warm with a side of low-FODMAP yogurt.

TIPS
*Check buying tips (see page 25).

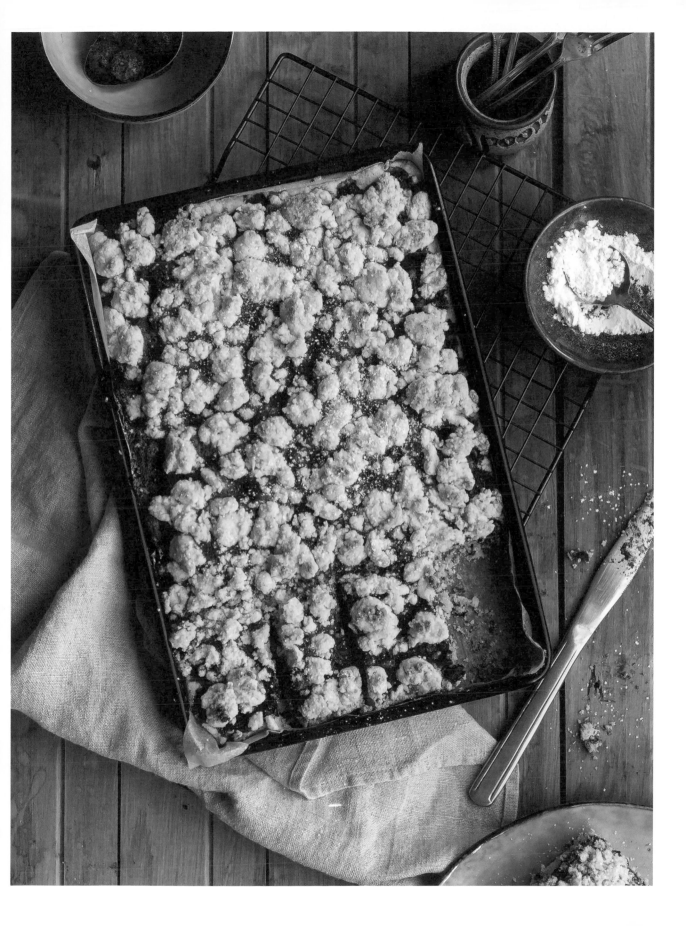

Dark Chocolate & Raspberry Brownie

PREP TIME: 35 minutes **COOK TIME**: 30 minutes
SERVES: 15

(LF) (GF) (DFO) (NF) (SF)

9 ounces (250g) dark chocolate

1¼ cups (250g) brown sugar

½ pound (2 sticks/250g) dairy-free spread or butter, cubed

4 large eggs

1 cup (140g) gluten-free self-rising flour*

6 tablespoons cocoa powder (GF if needed)

1½ teaspoons guar gum or xanthan gum

1½ cups (7oz/200g) fresh or frozen raspberries

This brownie is a decadent treat for the holiday season. It is perfect to take to parties, serve with Christmas dinner, or store in the freezer for unexpected guests.

1 Preheat oven to 350°F. Place the oven rack in the center of the oven. Line an 8-by-12-inch baking pan with parchment paper.

2 Heat the dark chocolate, brown sugar, and dairy-free spread or butter in a large saucepan over low heat. Melt, stirring continuously, until smooth and well combined. Remove from the heat, leave to cool for 3 minutes, then whisk in the eggs.

3 In a separate bowl, mix together the flour, cocoa powder, and gum.

4 Tip the dry ingredients into the melted chocolate mixture and stir until well combined. Fold in half of the raspberries.

5 Spoon the mixture into the prepared baking pan and spread evenly. Scatter the remaining raspberries over the top.

6 Bake in the preheated oven for 30 minutes. The top of the brownie should be spongy and shouldn't wobble too much. If the brownie is undercooked, bake for another 5–10 minutes.

7 Cool before slicing. This brownie should last for up to 3 days in an airtight container, or you can freeze it and serve it at a later date.

TIPS
*Check buying tips (see page 25).

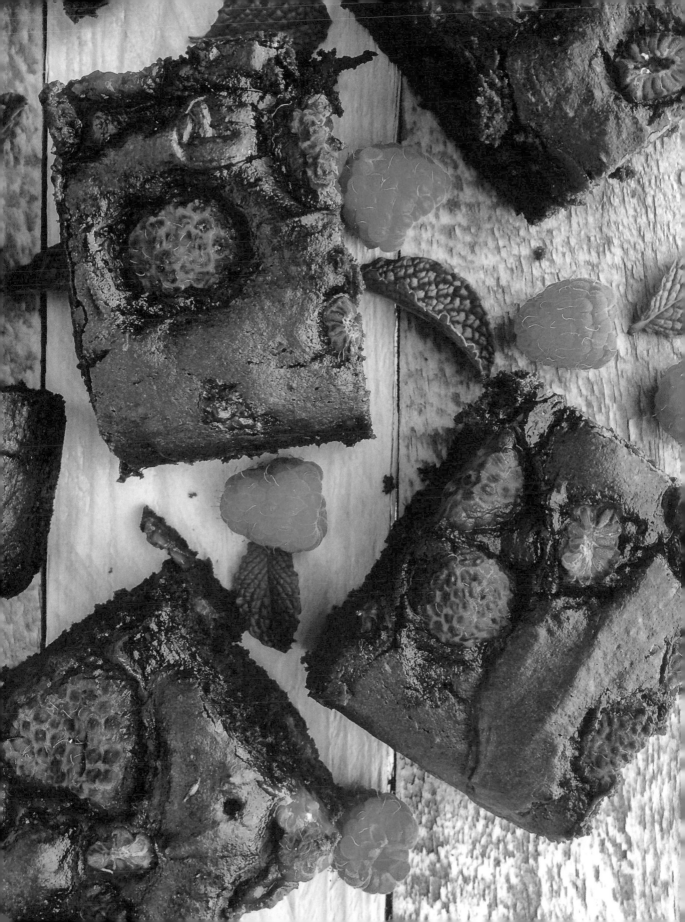

Dark Chocolate Chip Cookies

PREP TIME: 15 minutes **COOK TIME**: 12 minutes
MAKES: 24 cookies (limit 2 per serving)

(LF) (GF) (DFO) (NFO) (SF)

1¼ cups (175g) gluten-free all-purpose
   flour*
1½ tablespoons sunflower seed meal,
   almond meal, or hazelnut meal
¾ teaspoon baking soda (GF if
   needed)
Pinch of salt
½ cup (100g) firmly packed brown
   sugar
¼ cup (55g) white sugar
4 tablespoons dairy-free spread or
   butter (at room temperature)
3 tablespoons coconut oil, melted
1½ teaspoons vanilla essence
1 large egg + 1 egg yolk, lightly
   beaten
1 cup (6oz/170g) dark chocolate chips

When I was growing up, my mom made the best chocolate chip cookies. I'm keeping the family tradition going strong with these slightly chewy and oh-so-delicious low-FODMAP cookies. Enjoy two cookies per serving.

1 Preheat oven to 325°F. Place the oven rack in the center of the oven. Line a baking sheet with parchment paper.

2 In a large bowl, mix together the flour, sunflower seed or nut meal, baking soda, salt, brown sugar, and white sugar. Create a well in the middle of the dry ingredients and add the dairy-free spread or butter, coconut oil, vanilla essence, egg, and egg yolk. Mix until well combined. Then stir in the dark chocolate chips.

3 The dough should look glossy and hold together well. A tablespoon of dough should be just dry enough to handle and form into a soft ball. If the mixture is a little too wet, add another 1–2 tablespoons of flour.

4 Use a tablespoon to measure out the cookie dough, then gently shape into balls and flatten on the prepared baking sheet. Leave about 1 inch between each cookie.

5 Bake in the preheated oven for 10–12 minutes, until the bases of the cookies are slightly golden. Remove and leave to cool for 10 minutes before transferring to a wire rack.

TIPS
*Check buying tips (see page 25).

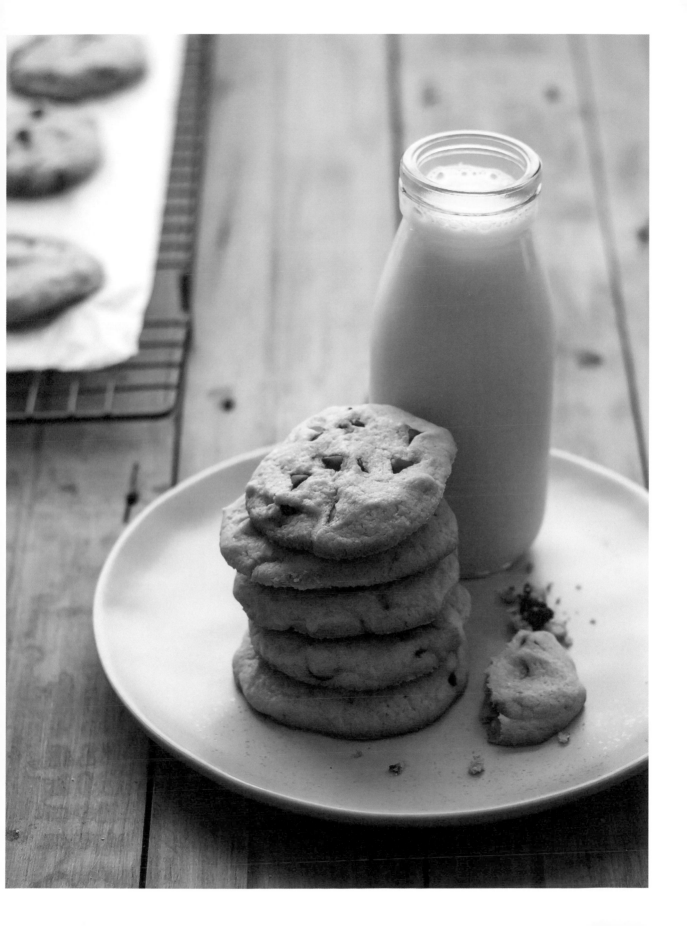

No-Bake Energy Bars

LF · GF · DFO · EF · NFO · SF

⅓ cup sunflower seed butter or
   peanut butter
6 tablespoons pure maple syrup
1½ cups puffed rice (GF if needed)
½ cup pumpkin seeds, roughly
   chopped
4 tablespoons dried cranberries,*
   roughly chopped
½ teaspoon ground ginger
½ teaspoon ground cinnamon
½ teaspoon guar gum or xanthan gum
   (optional)
1 ounce (30g) dark chocolate, roughly
   chopped (DF if needed)

These no-bake energy bars are so easy to make, and they are the perfect low-FODMAP grab-and-go snack! You can have these fully prepped and chilling in the fridge within 10 minutes.

1 Line an 8-inch square cake pan with parchment paper.

2 Melt the sunflower seed or peanut butter with the maple syrup in a large nonstick frying pan over medium–low heat. Once melted, turn off the heat and stir in all the remaining ingredients except the chocolate (the gum will make the slice less crumbly, but you don't have to use it). Once the ingredients are evenly coated in maple syrup, transfer the mixture to the pan.

3 Spread the mixture evenly in the pan. Place a piece of parchment paper on top and press the mixture firmly into the pan using your hands. If you don't compact the mixture firmly, the energy bars will crumble when you cut them.

4 In a small bowl, melt the chocolate in the microwave in 30-second bursts (stirring each time), until melted and smooth.

5 Remove the top layer of parchment paper and drizzle the mixture with melted chocolate.

6 Place in the fridge for 2 hours. Once cold, cut with a sharp knife. Store in an airtight container in the fridge or somewhere cool.

TIPS
These bars should remain fresh for about 2 weeks in the fridge, or you can pop them into the freezer and store for 2 months.

*Check buying tips (see page 25).

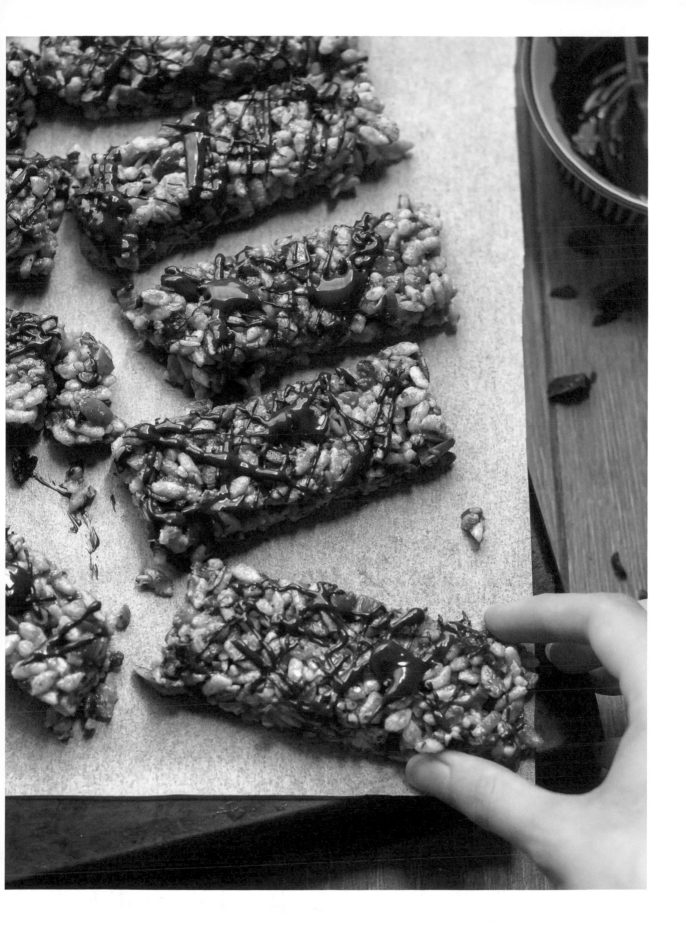

Dark Chocolate Truffle Balls

PREP TIME: 35 minutes **CHILL TIME**: 5 hours
MAKES: 30 truffle balls (limit 3 per serving)

(LF) (GFO) (DFO) (EF) (NF) (SF)

9 ounces (250g) dark chocolate (DF if needed)
2 tablespoons coconut oil, melted
1 teaspoon vanilla essence
1 tablespoon pure maple syrup
1 cup (250ml) canned coconut milk*
¼ cup dried shredded coconut
¼ cup sunflower and pumpkin seeds
¼ cup crushed gluten-free plain or vanilla cookies
2 tablespoons cocoa powder (GF if needed)

I love chocolate! These truffle balls make the perfect low-FODMAP treat. Just remember that they are chocolate heavy, which means they will only be as good as the quality of the chocolate you use.

1 Chop the dark chocolate into small pieces and place in a bowl with the coconut oil, vanilla essence, and maple syrup.

2 Heat the coconut milk in a small saucepan over low heat until it starts to steam, then pour onto the chocolate mixture. Mix gently with a spoon until well combined and smooth (do not whisk, as this will incorporate air into the mixture).

3 Cover the bowl with plastic wrap and leave to chill in the fridge for 4–5 hours (so the truffle mixture sets).

4 Just before you roll the truffles, toast the coconut in a small frying pan over medium heat for 1–2 minutes, until lightly golden. Toast the sunflower and pumpkin seeds for 2–3 minutes, until golden. Finely chop or crumble the coconut, seeds, and biscuits. Place the coatings in separate bowls.

5 Line a baking sheet with parchment paper. Wash your hands in very cold water (the colder your hands, the easier it is to roll the truffles). Using a teaspoon, scoop out truffle mixture and roll into balls in the palms of your hands before placing them on the baking sheet.

6 Decorate by rolling the balls through your choice of coating (coconut, seeds, biscuit crumbs, or cocoa powder). Return the truffles to the fridge for 30 minutes to firm up before serving.

TIPS
These truffles will last for a few days in the fridge.

*Check buying tips (see page 27).

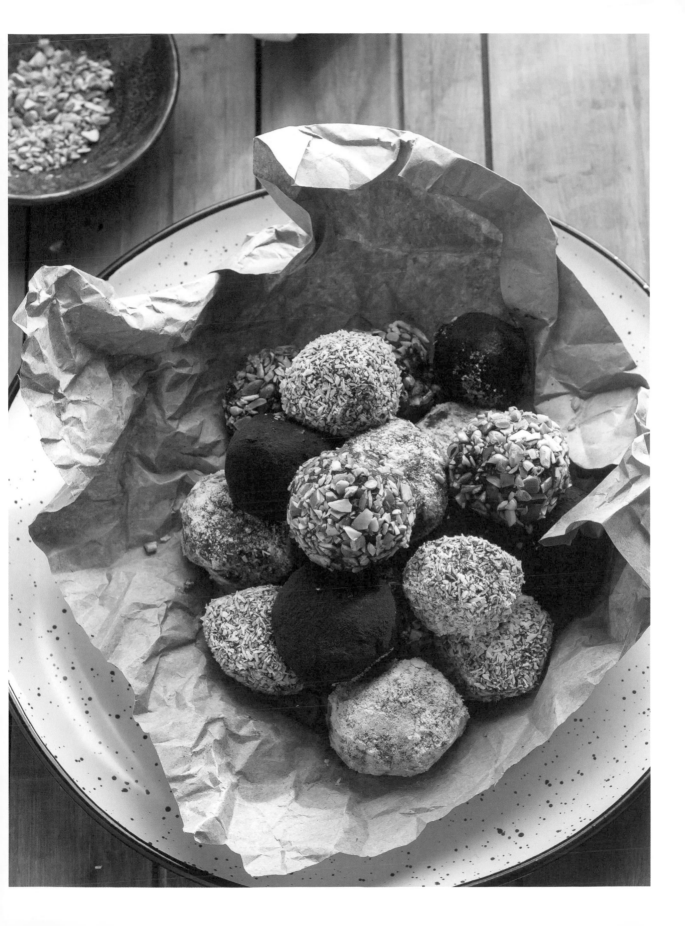

Lemon Meringue Pie

PREP TIME: 30 minutes + chilling time **COOK TIME**: 30 minutes
SERVES: 8–12

LF GF DFO NF SF

PASTRY

1¾ cups (240g) gluten-free all-purpose flour*

½ teaspoon guar gum or xanthan gum

8 tablespoons (1 stick/125g) dairy-free spread or butter

1 large egg, lightly beaten

1 tablespoon low-FODMAP milk*

1 egg yolk + 2 teaspoons low-FODMAP milk,* for glazing the pastry

LEMON CURD FILLING

2 large eggs

2 large egg yolks

½ cup (105g) white sugar

5 tablespoons (80g) dairy-free spread or butter

⅓ cup (85ml) freshly squeezed lemon juice

4 teaspoons lemon zest

3 tablespoons corn starch (GF if needed)

MERINGUE TOPPING

4 large egg whites (at room temperature)

1¼ cups (260g) superfine sugar

2 teaspoons corn starch (GF if needed)

TIPS

*Check buying tips (see pages 25–27).

I still remember the day I had my first bite of lemon meringue pie! I was in heaven. The lemon curd filling topped with soft marshmallow meringue was my idea of the best dessert ever.

1 Sift the flour and gum into a large bowl. Chop the dairy-free spread or butter into cubes (it should be as cold as possible), then rub it into the flour using your fingertips, until it resembles fine breadcrumbs. Add the egg and milk. Use your hands to bring the dough together and work it until smooth.

2 Pat the dough into a round, flat ball, roughly 1 inch thick. Wrap in plastic wrap and chill for at least 30 minutes (or overnight).

3 Preheat oven to 350°F. Grease a 9-inch tart pan.

4 Roll out the pastry on top of a piece of parchment paper until it is roughly ⅛ inch thick and 9 inches in diameter. If the pastry is crumbling, roll it out between two sheets of parchment paper. Carefully transfer the dough to the prepared tart pan. Firmly press any cracks back together. Trim away any overhanging pastry and prick the base with a fork.

5 To blind-bake the pastry, cover the pastry with parchment paper. Pour dried rice or dried beans on top of the paper to hold it down evenly.

6 Bake in the preheated oven for 10–12 minutes. Remove the parchment paper and rice or beans and bake the pastry for another 5 minutes. Remove from the oven and brush with egg yolk and milk, then bake for another 5–10 minutes until lightly golden. Leave to cool for 30 minutes (it should be just warmer than room temperature before filling).

CONTINUED ON PAGE 170

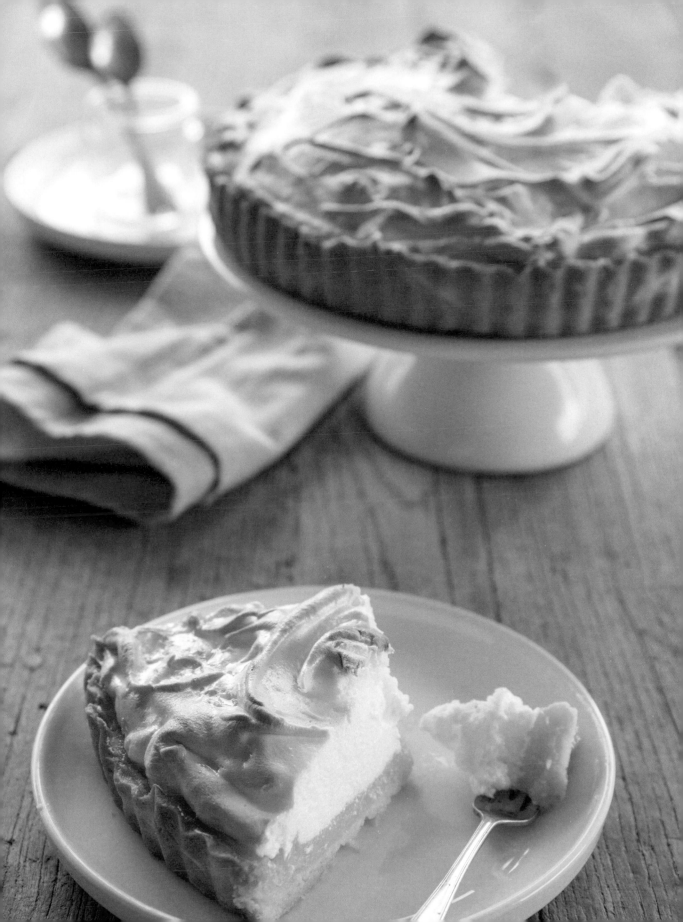

- Make sure you blind-bake the pastry until it is golden and firm to the touch.

- Allow the pastry and lemon curd filling to cool to about room temperature before assembling the pie.

- Weigh the egg whites. The ratio should be 2 parts sugar to 1 part egg whites.

- Make sure the meringue is smooth and that the sugar has fully dissolved into the egg whites during whisking.

7 While the piecrust bakes, make the lemon curd filling. Place the whole eggs, egg yolks, and white sugar in a small saucepan. Whisk until well combined and smooth. Place over low heat and add the dairy-free spread or butter and the lemon juice and zest, stirring continuously until the spread has melted. Turn the heat up to medium. Continue to cook and stir until the mixture thickens (this should take 5–7 minutes).

8 Dissolve the corn starch in ½ cup of warm water and mix. Allow to thicken for another 2 minutes. It's done when it "plops" off the spoon. Leave to cool for 30 minutes.

9 Preheat oven to 325°F.

10 Once the piecrust and lemon curd filling have cooled, use an egg beater to whip the egg whites until they form stiff peaks. As the eggs whip, gently pour in half of the sugar, 1 tablespoon at a time. Next, gently fold in the corn starch. Continue to beat in the remaining sugar, 1 tablespoon at a time until glossy, thick, and stiff peaks form.

11 Pour the lemon curd filling into the piecrust, then immediately top with the meringue.

12 Bake in the preheated oven for 10–15 minutes, until the meringue is golden brown (watch closely as the meringue can brown quickly).

13 Leave to cool fully before slicing.

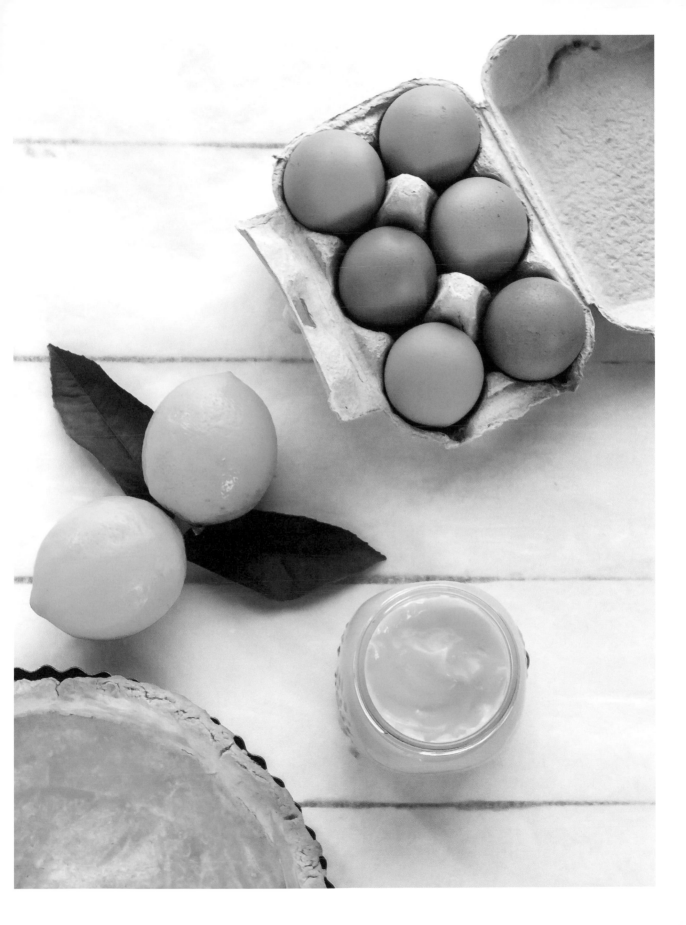

Berry Nice Pavlova

PREP TIME: 30 minutes **COOK TIME:** 45 minutes + 2 hours rest time
SERVES: 8

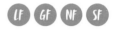

PAVLOVA

6 large egg whites
1½ cups (315g) superfine sugar
1 teaspoon lemon juice
¼ teaspoon salt
2 teaspoons corn starch (GF if needed)

RASPBERRY REDUCTION

¼ cup (1oz/30g) chopped raspberries
1 tablespoon superfine sugar
1 teaspoon lemon juice
2 tablespoons water
½ teaspoon corn starch (GF if
    needed), dissolved in 1 tablespoon
    cold water

BERRY TOPPINGS

1 cup (250ml) cream
½ teaspoon vanilla essence
2 cups (8½oz/250g) strawberries
1 cup (4½oz/125g) blueberries
1 cup (4½oz/125g) raspberries
Small handful of baby mint leaves

Pavlova is a Kiwi classic and I adore its fluffy marshmallow center. Make it low FODMAP by topping it with fresh strawberries, blueberries, and raspberries.

1 Preheat oven to 300°F. Place the oven rack in the center of the oven. Draw a 7-by-12-inch rectangle on a sheet of parchment paper and place it facing down on a baking sheet. Make sure your bowl and beaters are completely clean of residual fat or grease (otherwise the egg whites won't whip).

2 Using electric beaters or a cake mixer, beat the egg whites until they form foamy, soft peaks (the beaters should leave a trail as you lift them up). Next, starting at a low speed, slowly spoon in the superfine sugar, leaving a few seconds between each spoonful.

3 Increase the speed of the beaters and continue to beat the egg whites until they form stiff peaks. They should be glossy and hold their shape when you lift up the beaters. (You will need to beat the mixture for longer than you think for stiff peaks.)

4 Fold in the lemon juice, salt, and corn starch.

5 Scoop the mixture into the middle of the parchment paper and shape into the rectangle. Decorate the top by making swirls with a knife.

6 Place the baking sheet in the middle of the oven and turn the heat down to 250°F. Bake for 45 minutes. When the pavlova is done it should look pale and dry, and a toothpick inserted into the middle should come out with a thick, sticky marshmallow coating. Turn the oven off and leave the pavlova in the oven for 1–2 hours with the door ajar.

CONTINUED ON PAGE 174

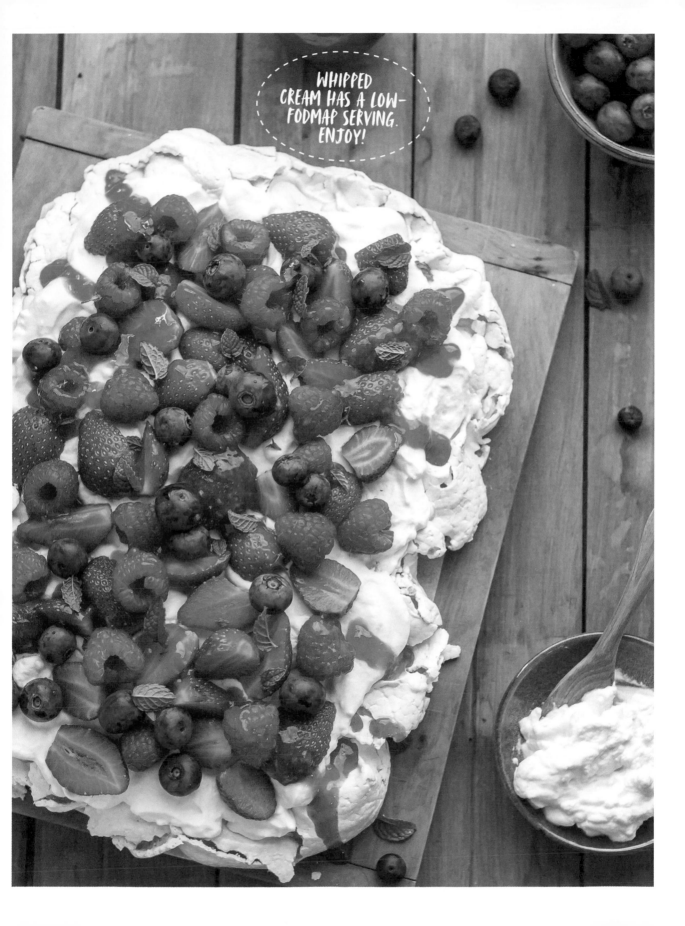

WHIPPED CREAM HAS A LOW-FODMAP SERVING. ENJOY!

7 Make the raspberry reduction by mixing the chopped raspberries, sugar, lemon juice, and water together in a small saucepan. Simmer over medium heat until the sugar dissolves. Stir in the corn starch mixture. Remove the reduction from the heat once it drizzles nicely from a spoon (if it becomes too thick, just add more water).

8 Just before serving, beat the cream until it is soft and fluffy, and fold in the vanilla essence.

9 Top the pavlova with the whipped cream, scatter with the berries, and drizzle with the raspberry reduction. Garnish with a handful of baby mint leaves.

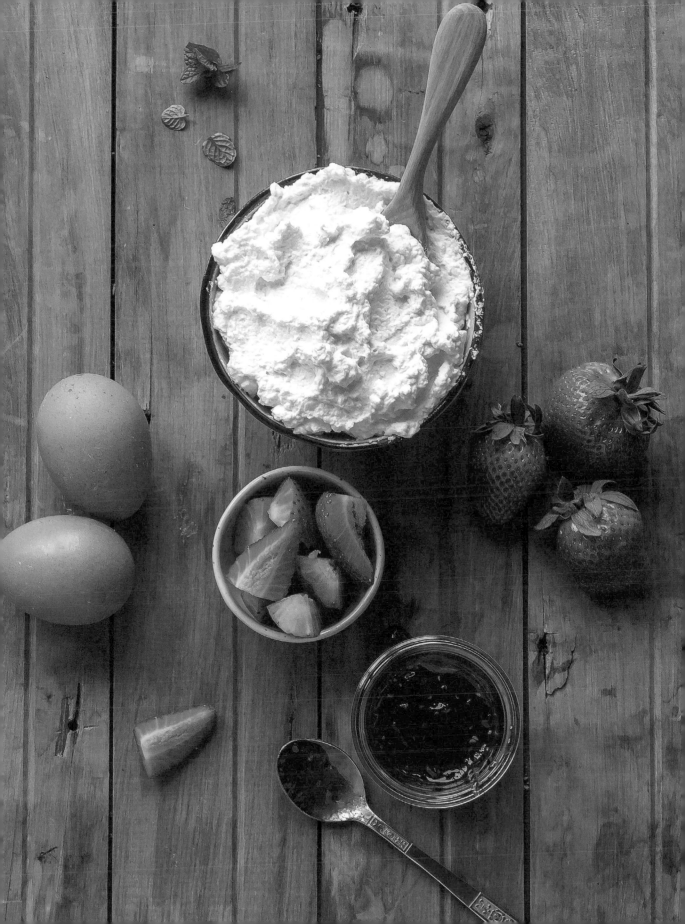

Strawberry & Banana Ice Cream with Chocolate Fudge Sauce

PREP TIME: 15 minutes + chilling time
SERVES: 4

(LF) (GF) (DFO) (EF) (NF) (SF)

2 small (5½oz/160g) frozen bananas
   (no brown spots)
2½ cups (10½oz/300g) frozen
   strawberries
5 tablespoons coconut yogurt*
2 tablespoons pure maple syrup
1 teaspoon vanilla essence
Chocolate Fudge Sauce (see recipe on
   page 217)

It's easy, it's delicious, and it's simple! This strawberry banana ice cream goes brilliantly with chocolate fudge sauce.

1 Chop the frozen bananas and strawberries into small pieces. Place in a food processor with the coconut yogurt, maple syrup, and vanilla essence. Blend, and scrape down the sides of the food processor as needed, until smooth (this will take 5 minutes or so).

2 Taste and add more maple syrup or vanilla essence if desired.

3 Serve immediately as soft serve (if you're impatient!) or freeze for a couple of hours until slightly firm. Top with Chocolate Fudge Sauce.

TIPS

Avoid using overripe bananas as they are higher FODMAP and the banana flavor will be very strong.

Make sure you freeze the bananas and strawberries in advance as this helps give the ice cream a better texture.

*Check buying tips (see page 25).

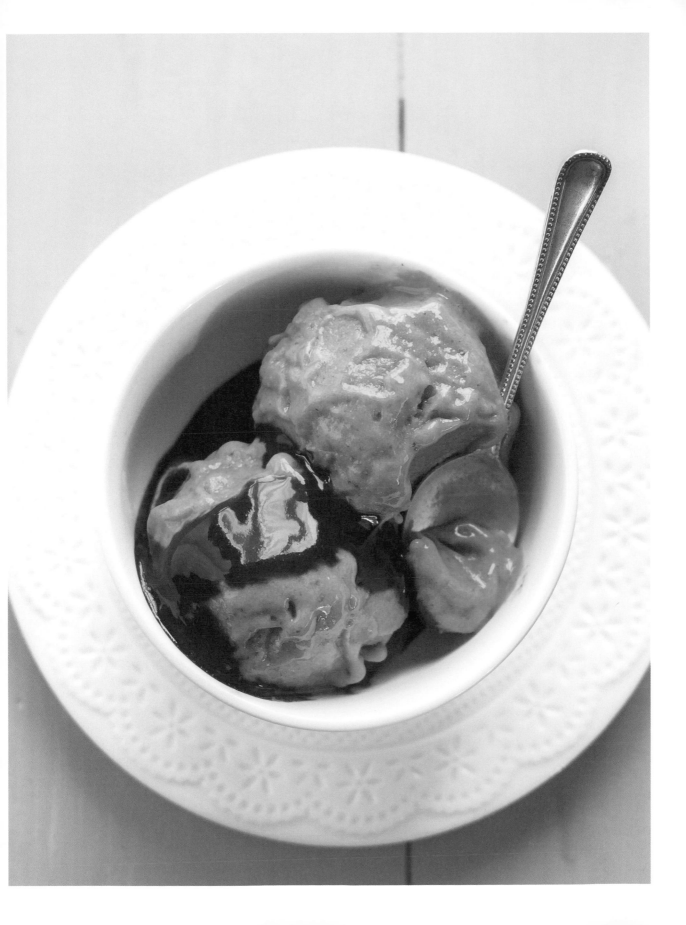

Banana Butterscotch Pudding

PREP TIME: 15 minutes **COOK TIME:** 45 minutes
SERVES: 6

(LF) (GF) (DFO) (EFO) (NF) (SF)

1⅓ cups (190g) gluten-free all-purpose
   flour*
3 teaspoons baking powder (GF if
   needed)
1 cup (7oz/200g) mashed firm banana
   (no brown spots)
1 large egg, beaten
1 teaspoon vanilla essence
½ cup (125ml) low-FODMAP milk*
6 tablespoons (100g) dairy-free spread
   or butter, melted

BUTTERSCOTCH SAUCE

½ cup (100g) lightly packed brown
   sugar
1 tablespoon corn starch (GF if
   needed)
2 cups (500ml) boiling water
1 tablespoon dark molasses
2 tablespoons pure maple syrup

TIPS

To make this recipe egg free,
you can replace the egg with a
commercial egg replacer. I used
the equivalent of two eggs' worth
of the replacer.

*Check buying tips (see pages
25–27).

Feel like something sweet? Then this banana butterscotch
pudding is the perfect comfort dessert. It combines the flavor
of banana bread with the gooey goodness of butterscotch
sauce.

1 Preheat oven to 350°F. Place the oven rack in the center of
the oven. Grease an 11-by-8-inch ovenproof baking dish.

2 Mix the flour and baking powder in a large mixing bowl.
Add the banana, egg, vanilla essence, milk, and dairy-free
spread or butter, and mix until well combined. Spoon into the
prepared dish.

3 Combine the brown sugar and corn starch in a small bowl.
Sprinkle evenly over the pudding mixture.

4 In a medium bowl, mix together the boiling water,
molasses, and maple syrup. Gently pour over the pudding
(pour onto the back of a dessert spoon to disperse the liquid).

5 Bake in the preheated oven for 30–40 minutes, until a
toothpick inserted into the center of the pudding comes out
clean and the top is golden brown. It's okay if the pudding is
wobbly.

MOLASSES IS LOW FODMAP IN SMALL SERVINGS. AVOID LARGER SERVINGS AS THEY BECOME HIGH FODMAP.

Dark Chocolate Self-Saucing Pudding

PREP TIME: 10 minutes **COOK TIME:** 15 minutes
SERVES: 4–6

(LF) (GF) (DFO) (EFO) (NFO) (SF)

BASE

½ cup (70g) gluten-free all-purpose flour*

1 tablespoon sunflower seed meal,
    almond meal, or hazelnut meal

¼ cup (50g) firmly packed brown sugar

2 teaspoons baking powder (GF if
    needed)

2½ tablespoons cocoa powder (GF if
    needed)

½ cup (125ml) low-FODMAP milk*

2 tablespoons dairy-free spread or
    butter, melted

1 large egg, lightly beaten

1 teaspoon vanilla essence

2 ounces (50g) dark chocolate, finely
    chopped

TOPPING

1 tablespoon cocoa powder (GF if
    needed)

¼ cup (50g) firmly packed brown sugar

1 cup (250ml) boiling water

TIPS

I have a nut allergy, so I used
sunflower seed meal that I made at
home by blending sunflower seeds
in a food processor. You can replace
this ingredient with almond meal or
hazelnut meal if you prefer.

To make this recipe egg free,
you can replace the egg with a
commercial egg replacer.

*Check buying tips (see pages
25–27).

I'm a self-confessed chocolate addict! Indulging in a gooey chocolate pudding is always the perfect way to lift my spirits after a bad day. This recipe is super easy and a great way to get kids into the kitchen.

1 Preheat oven to 350°F. Place the oven rack in the center of the oven. Grease an 8-inch square ovenproof baking dish.

2 Place the flour, sunflower seed or nut meal, brown sugar, baking powder, and cocoa powder in a large bowl and mix until well combined.

3 In a separate bowl, mix together the milk, dairy-free spread or butter, egg, and vanilla. Stir the wet mixture through the dry mixture and spoon into the baking dish, spreading the mixture evenly. Sprinkle the chocolate on top.

4 Mix together the cocoa powder and brown sugar for the topping. Sprinkle over the pudding, then gently pour the boiling water in (pour onto the back of a dessert spoon to disperse the water).

5 Bake in the preheated oven for 15 minutes, until the top is firm and a toothpick comes out relatively clean.

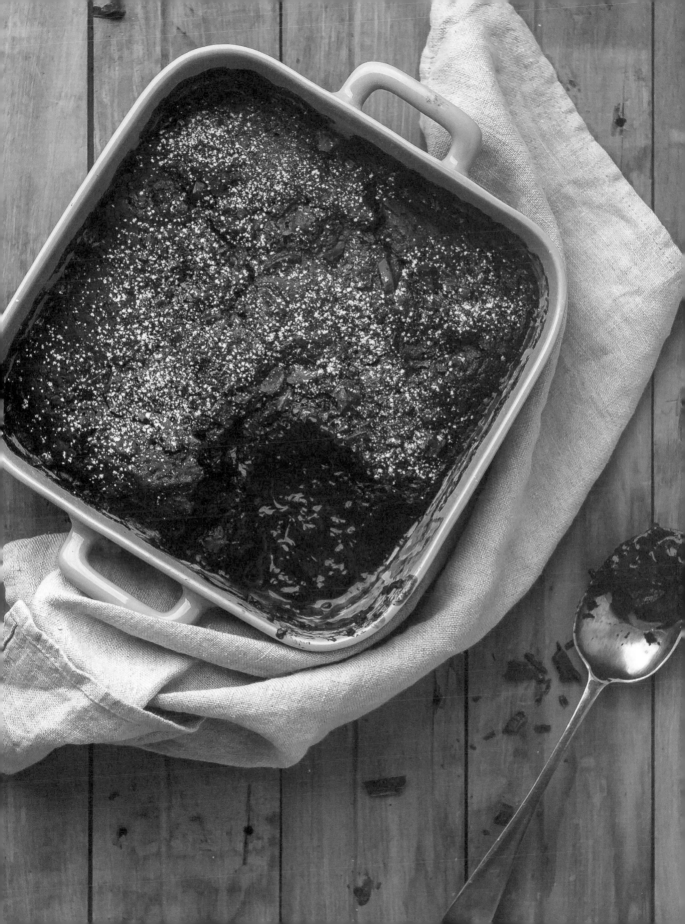

Mini Strawberry & Rhubarb Crumbles

PREP TIME: 10 minutes **COOK TIME**: 20 minutes
SERVES: 3

(LF) (GF) (DFO) (EF) (NF) (SF)

1 cup (4½oz/130g) chopped fresh
   rhubarb, washed and cut into small
   pieces
2 tablespoons water
1½ teaspoons white sugar
1 cup (5oz/140g) fresh or frozen
   strawberries, halved
1 tablespoon corn starch (GF if
   needed)

CRUMBLE
1 cup gluten-free cornflakes*
¼ cup (50g) brown sugar
¼ cup (35g) gluten-free all-purpose
   flour*
3 tablespoons dried shredded coconut
2 tablespoons pumpkin seeds
4 tablespoons dairy-free spread or
   butter

These mini crumbles make a delicious dessert. The crumble
is yummy by itself, or you can serve it with low-FODMAP
ice cream or yogurt.

1 Preheat oven to 400°F. Place the oven rack in the center of
the oven. Grease three small ramekins.

2 Place the rhubarb in a small, shallow roasting pan with the
water. Sprinkle with 1 teaspoon of the white sugar. Roast for
10 minutes, until tender. Then remove and turn the oven down
to 350°F.

3 While the rhubarb roasts, make the crumble in a large
bowl. Crush the cornflakes and mix together with the brown
sugar, flour, coconut, and pumpkin seeds.

4 Soften but do not melt the dairy-free spread or butter. Add
to the dry ingredients and work into the mixture until it forms
small crumbs and there are no large lumps left.

5 Divide the rhubarb among the ramekins. Add the
strawberries and sprinkle with the corn starch and remaining
white sugar. Spread the crumble topping evenly on top. Place
the dishes on a flat baking sheet.

6 Bake in the preheated oven for 15–20 minutes, or until the
topping is golden brown. Serve hot.

TIPS
*Check buying tips (see page 25).

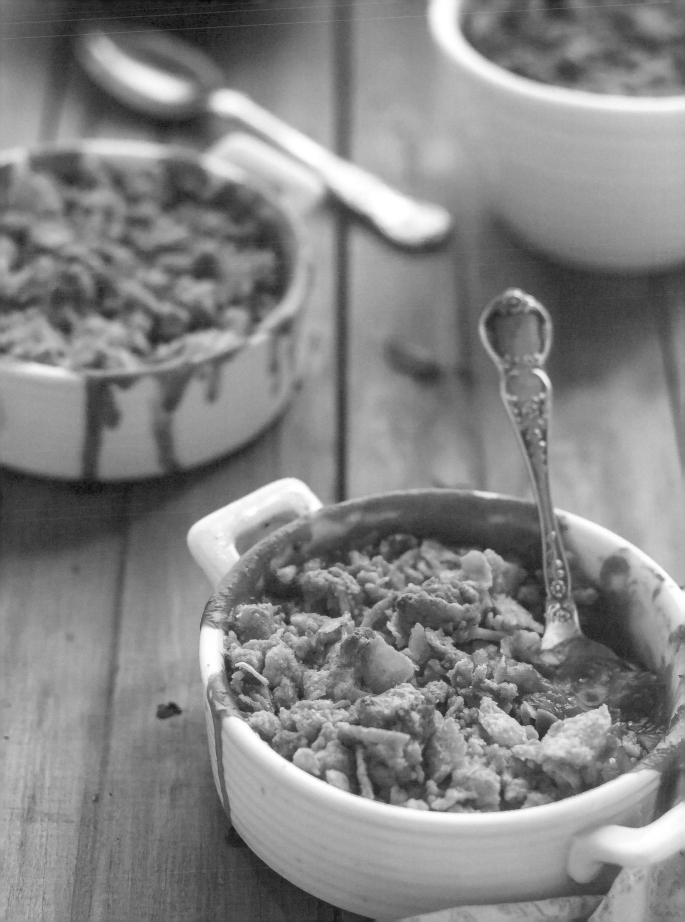

Berry Bliss Frozen Yogurt Bark

PREP TIME: 5 minutes + freezing time
SERVES: 6

(LF) (GF) (DFO) (EF) (NF) (SF)

5 fresh or frozen strawberries

1 teaspoon vanilla essence

1¼ cup (300ml) lactose-free or
   coconut yogurt*

2 tablespoons strawberry jam

15 fresh or frozen blueberries

8 fresh or frozen raspberries

There is nothing better than a frozen treat! And this bark, made from low-FODMAP yogurt and berries, is one of my favorites. This recipe takes only 5 minutes to prepare but you will need to freeze the bark for 2–3 hours before eating.

1 Line a small baking sheet with parchment paper. Chop the strawberries into small bite-sized pieces.

2 Mix the vanilla essence in the yogurt.

3 Spoon the yogurt onto the baking sheet and spread using a flat knife until it is about ⅓ inch thick. Make sure the yogurt is thick enough to push the fruit into.

4 Melt the strawberry jam in the microwave in 10-second bursts, then swirl into the yogurt using a spoon.

5 Sprinkle the strawberries and blueberries over the yogurt and crumble the raspberries on top.

6 Freeze for 2–3 hours until hard. Cut using a sharp knife. Store in an airtight container in the freezer.

TIPS
*Check buying tips (see page 25).

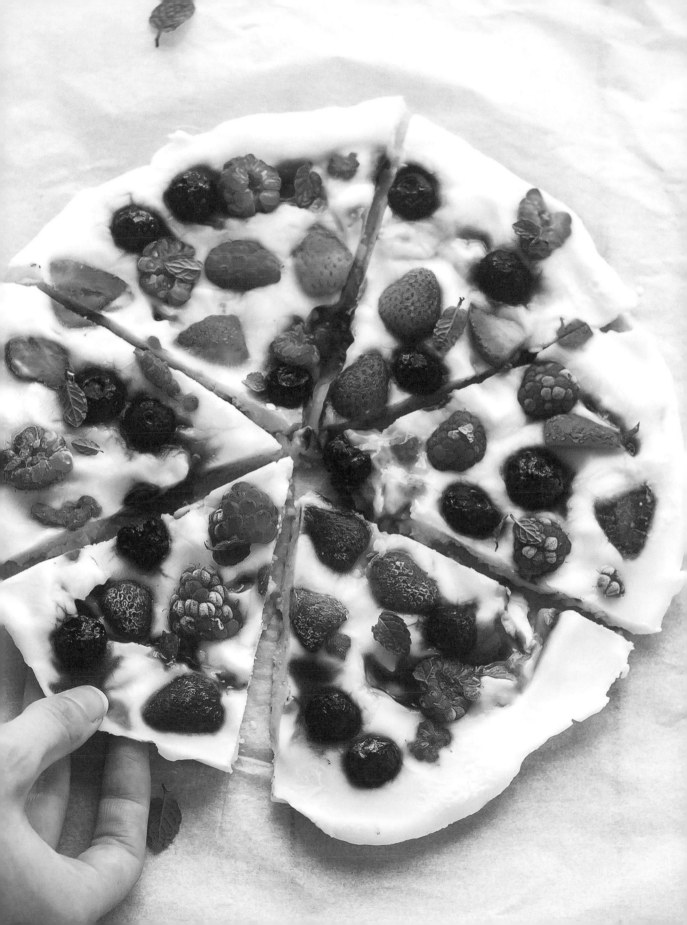

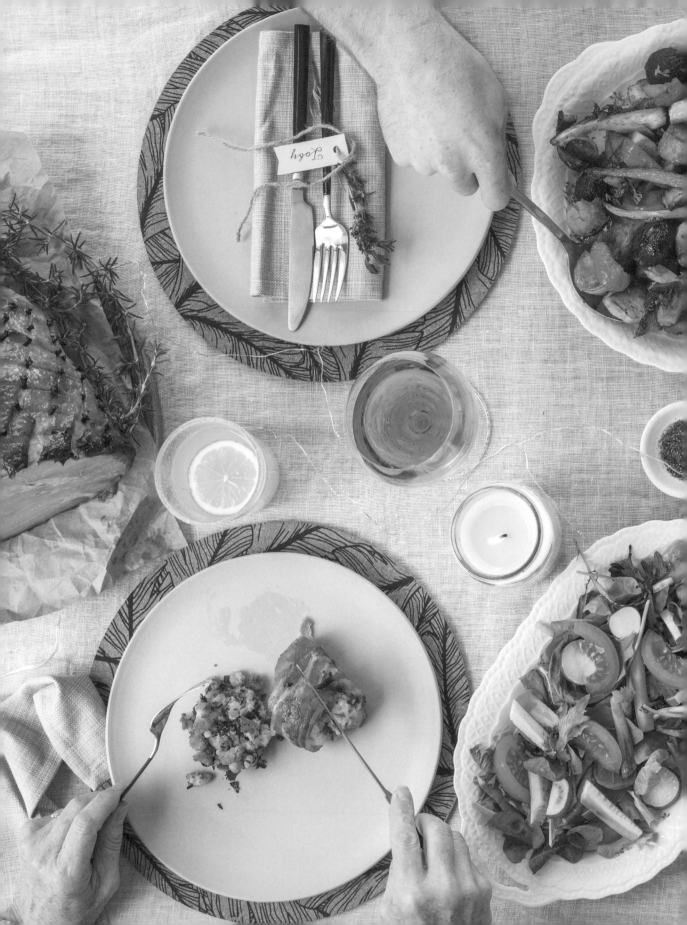

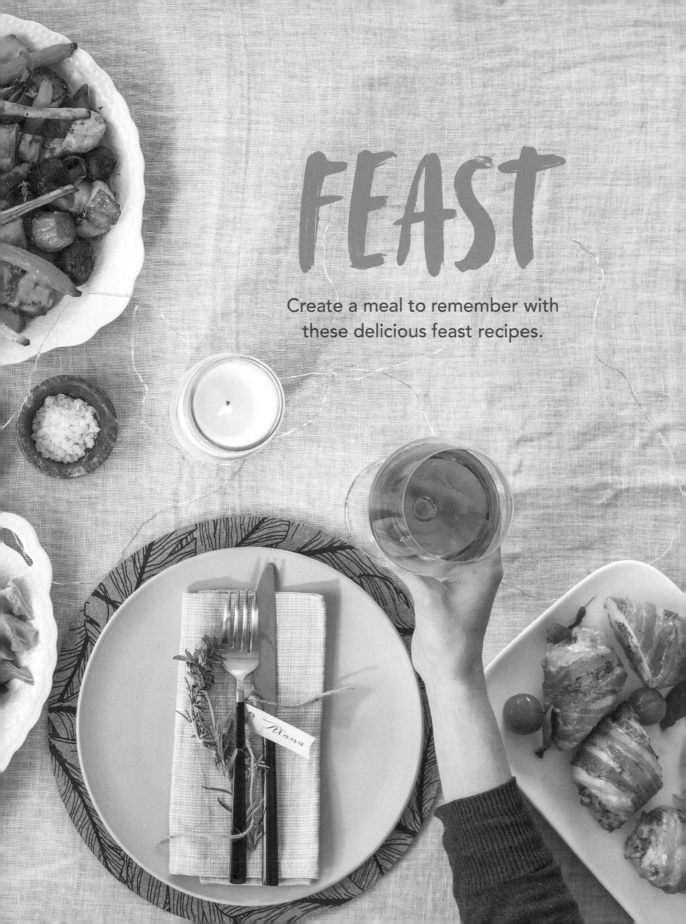

FEAST

Create a meal to remember with
these delicious feast recipes.

Antipasto Platter

Kick off your low-FODMAP gathering with an antipasto platter. Choose a mixture of platter options, then let your guests mix and match!

CHEESE
- Camembert
- Brie
- blue cheese
- Pecorino-style cheese
- feta

CRACKERS & BREAD
- plain rice crackers
- crostini made from toasted low-FODMAP bread brushed with garlic-infused oil

MEATS
- salami*
- plain smoked salmon
- smoked chicken*
- plain shaved ham (no honey)

DIPS
- Traditional Hummus (see page 210)
- Easy Basil Pesto (see page 215)

OTHER OPTIONS
- veggie sticks (carrot, red bell pepper, cucumber)
- cherry tomatoes
- fresh fruit (grapes, blueberries, strawberries, raspberries, sliced kiwifruit, sliced pineapple)
- olives (green or black, pitted)
- sundried tomatoes (low-FODMAP serving is 2 pieces)
- thinly sliced red or green chile

TIPS
*Check that they don't contain onion or garlic.

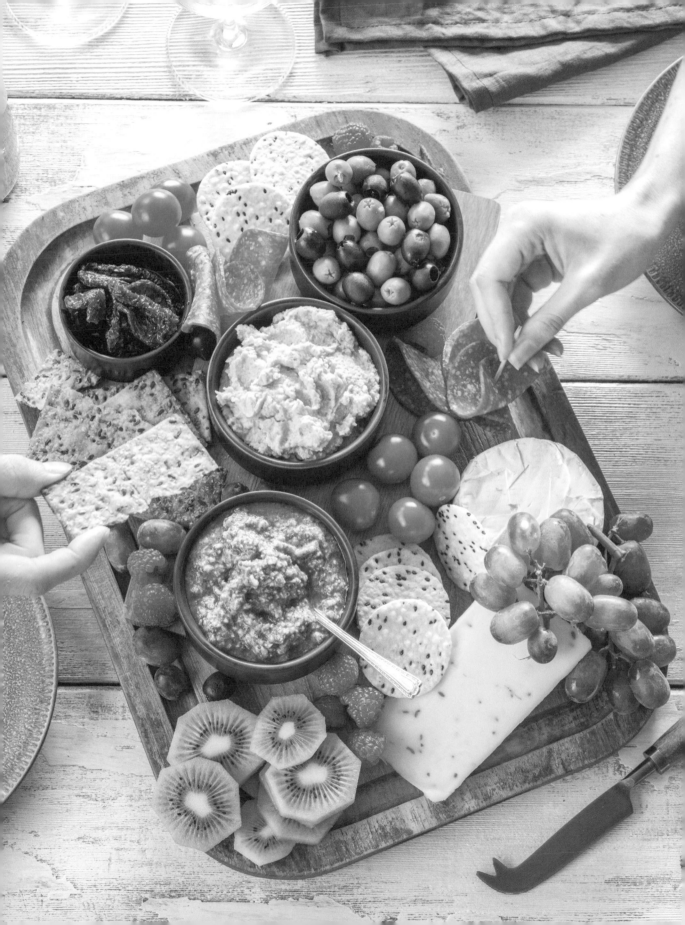

Pork Loin Roast with Herb Rice Stuffing

PREP TIME: 1 hour COOK TIME: 2 hours
SERVES: 10

LF GF DF EF NF SF

1½ cups (4oz/120g) chopped leeks
(green leaves only)
1 tablespoon each of olive oil and
garlic-infused oil*
1 cup arborio rice
About 2 cups (500ml) low-FODMAP
chicken stock* (GF if needed)
1 cup chopped fresh parsley
¼ cup finely chopped scallions (green
leaves only)
1 teaspoon dried oregano
½ teaspoon dried thyme
3 tablespoons pumpkin seeds
5½ pounds (2.5kg) pork loin roast
Drizzle of olive oil
A few grinds of rock salt

TIPS

If possible, take the stuffing to the
butcher and ask them to stuff and
tie the pork loin roast for you. Ask
them to score the skin and fat for
you as well.

*Check buying tips (see pages
25–26).

This delicious recipe makes enough to feed a small army and
is well worth the effort. The pork is juicy, the skin is crunchy,
and the rice stuffing is packed full of herby goodness.

1   In a large saucepan over medium heat, fry the leeks in
the oils for 2 minutes. Add the rice and stir for 1 minute. Add
½ cup chicken stock at a time, stirring often until the liquid
has been absorbed. Continue adding and stirring in the stock
(turn the heat down if necessary). Once the rice has absorbed
2 cups of stock (this should take about 20 minutes), check to
see if it is cooked. If it isn't, add more stock and continue to
cook. When cooked, the rice should be tender and sticky but
not too wet.

2   Remove the rice from the heat and stir in the parsley,
scallions, oregano, thyme, and pumpkin seeds. Transfer to a
plastic container or bowl and leave to cool.

3   Stuff the pork with the herb rice stuffing, roll up, and secure
with string.

4   Preheat oven to 425°F.

5   Rub the pork skin with olive oil and season generously with
salt. Place in a roasting pan and roast for 30 minutes. Remove
from the oven and baste with the pork juices (drizzle the pork
juices over the roast). Lightly season again with salt.

6   Turn the oven down to 400°F and roast the pork for about
another 1½ hours. Baste the pork every 30 minutes. If the skin
looks like it might burn, cover it with foil.

7   Remove the pork from the oven when the skin is golden
and the juices run clear (insert a sharp knife into the roast).
Rest for 10 minutes before carving.

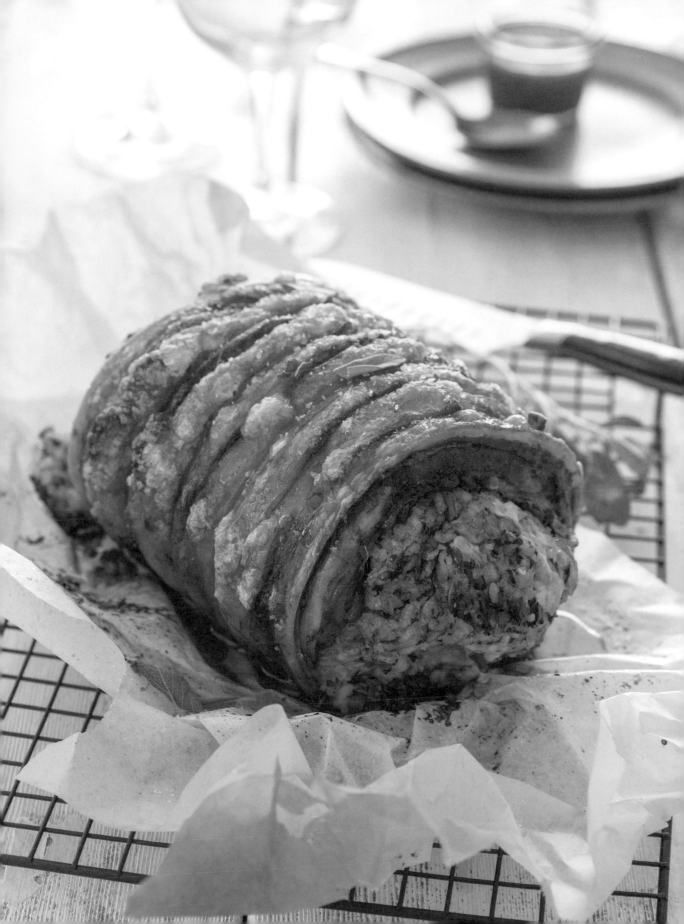

Maple-Glazed Ham

PREP TIME: 30 minutes **COOK TIME:** 1½ hours
SERVES: 25

(LF) (GF) (DF) (EF) (NF) (SF)

1 (18lb/8kg) ham on the bone
⅓ cup (85ml) pure maple syrup
⅓ cup (65g) firmly packed brown
    sugar
⅓ cup (85ml) freshly squeezed orange
    juice (1–2 large oranges)
1 tablespoon Dijon mustard*
30 whole cloves

There are plenty of ways to create a low-FODMAP glazed ham this holiday season without using honey. I love using brown sugar, maple syrup, freshly squeezed orange juice, and cloves to create a tender and juicy ham.

1 Preheat oven to 300°F. Place the oven rack at the lowest level in the oven. Line a large roasting pan with two layers of parchment paper.

2 Place the ham in the prepared roasting pan and bake for 10 minutes (this will help warm the skin and make it easier to remove).

3 While the ham warms, whisk together the maple syrup, brown sugar, orange juice, and Dijon mustard to make the glaze.

4 Remove the ham from the oven and increase the oven temperature to 350°F. Make a cut around the shank of the ham (about 3½ inches from the skinny end), using a sharp knife. Run the knife under the rind around the edge of the ham, then gently run your fingers back and forth between the rind and the fat to separate. You should then be able to gently lift off the rind in one piece. Discard.

5 Score the fat in a diamond pattern, about ¼ inch deep. Stud the centers of the diamonds with cloves. Baste with one-third of the glaze.

6 Bake in the preheated oven for 1½ hours, brushing with glaze every 25 minutes. Remove from the oven once the fat has turned a deep golden brown.

TIPS
*Check buying tips (see page 26).

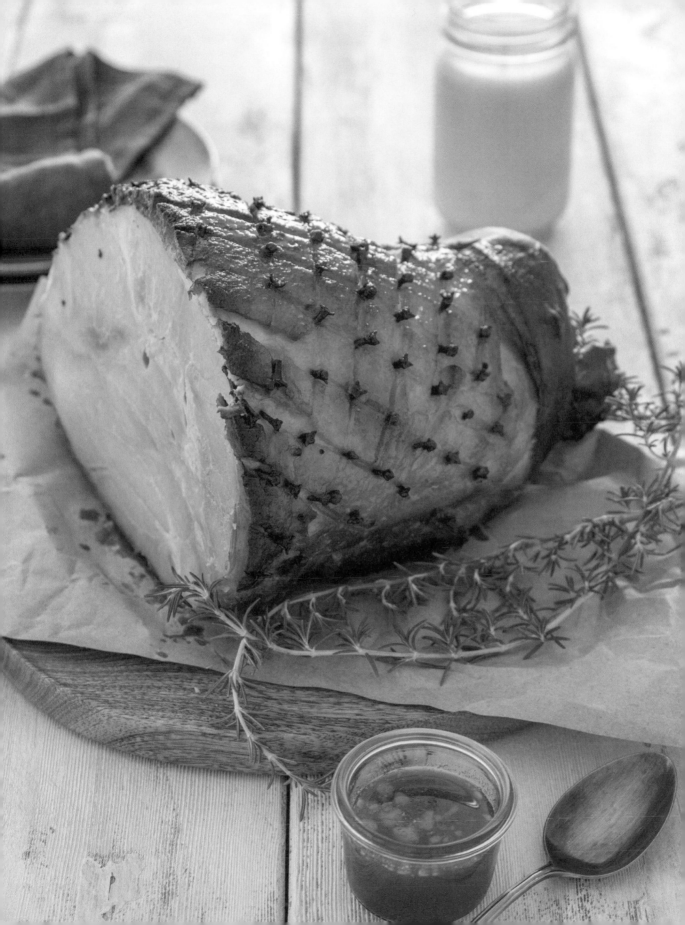

Crunchy Herb Stuffing

PREP TIME: 10 minutes **COOK TIME**: 20 minutes
SERVES: 12

(LF) (GFO) (DFO) (EF) (NF) (SF)

10 slices low-FODMAP or gluten-free
   bread,* shredded into small pieces
4 tablespoons dairy-free spread or
   butter, melted
1 tablespoon garlic-infused oil*
1½ cups (4oz/120g) chopped leeks
   (green leaves only)
Large handful of fresh parsley, finely
   chopped
1 teaspoon dried sage
1 teaspoon dried oregano
½ teaspoon dried thyme
¼ teaspoon sea salt
¼ teaspoon black pepper
½ cup (125ml) low-FODMAP chicken
   or vegetable stock* (GF if needed)

I love this stuffing! Crunchy on the outside, soft and moist on
the inside. The great thing about this recipe is you can make
the stuffing the day before and just pop it in the oven to cook
for 10 minutes as your roast rests. Enjoy!

1 Preheat oven to 350°F. Spray or grease a 12-hole muffin
pan with oil.

2 In a large bowl, toss together the bread, dairy-free spread
or butter, and oil. Once the bread is well coated, spread it on a
baking sheet and bake for 5 minutes. Turn the bread and cook
for another 3–5 minutes, until it starts turning golden brown,
then remove from the oven.

3 I like my stuffing chunky and crunchy; however, if you want
a finer stuffing, blitz it in a food processor.

4 Return the toasted bread to the bowl and mix in all the
remaining ingredients except the stock. (You can do this in
advance, then store in the fridge until you are ready to use.)

5 Heat the stock until hot, then mix in the stuffing mix—it
should be moist but not soggy (you can add more stock if
needed). Spoon the mixture into the prepared muffin pan until
the holes are completely full, then press down lightly.

6 Bake in the preheated oven for 10–15 minutes, until the
tops are crunchy. Serve hot with a drizzle of homemade gravy.

TIPS
*Check buying tips (see pages
25–26).

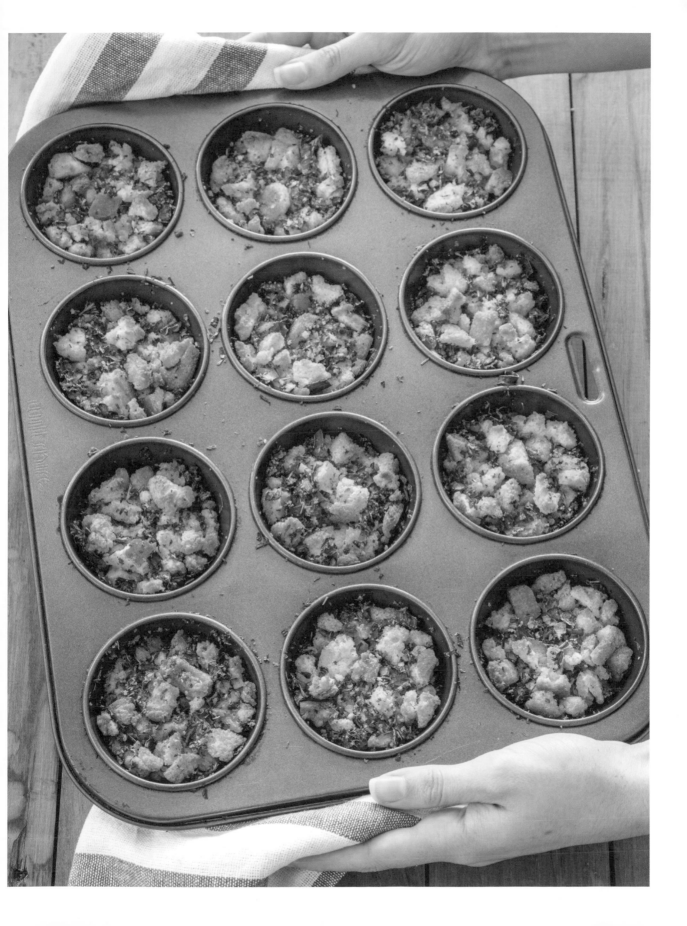

Pesto-Stuffed Chicken Breasts Wrapped in Bacon

PREP TIME: 25 minutes **COOK TIME:** 40 minutes
SERVES: 8

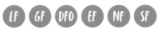

1¾ pounds (800g) chicken breast fillets

½ cup Easy Basil Pesto (see recipe on page 215)

¾ cup (3oz/85g) grated Cheddar or vegan cheese*

A few grinds of salt and pepper, to taste

8 slices bacon*

There are no leftovers when these chicken breasts are on the menu! They are always a hit at my winter feasts. Just remember: this dish is rich, so make sure you serve it with plenty of side dishes.

1 Preheat oven to 400°F.

2 Remove chicken skin and pound fillets until they are ½ inch thick.

3 Spread the pesto over the chicken and cover with cheese. Season with salt and pepper. Roll up each chicken breast and wrap with bacon. Secure with a toothpick.

4 Place a wire baking rack in a roasting pan. Place the rolled chicken on the rack and bake in the preheated oven for 30–40 minutes, until the juices run clear.

5 Grill for 3–4 minutes until the bacon is crispy.

6 Leave to rest for 5 minutes, then slice and serve.

TIPS
*Check buying tips (see pages 25–26).

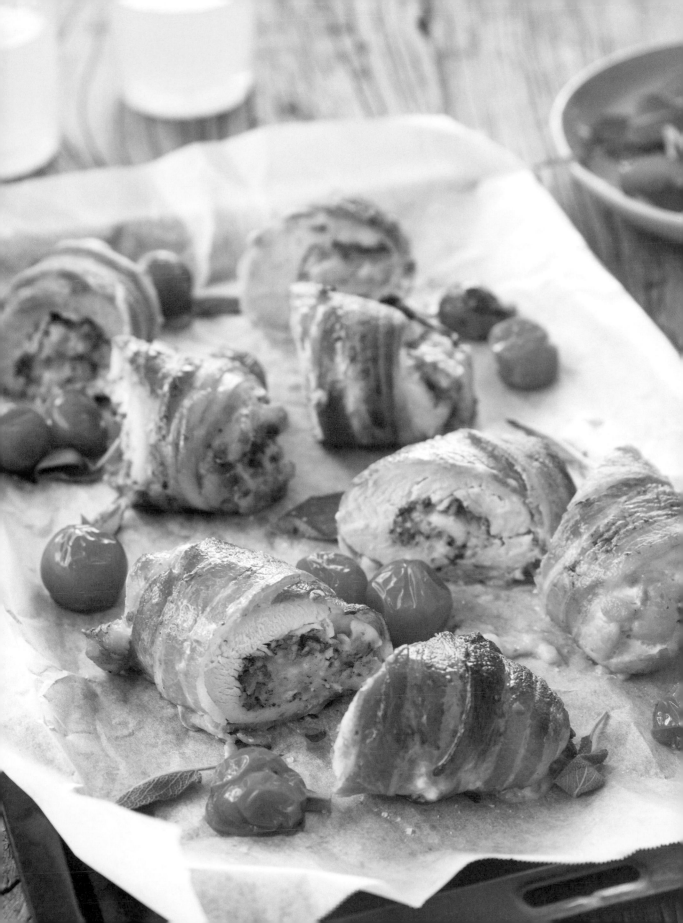

Gorgeous Roasted Veggies

PREP TIME: 15 minutes **COOK TIME**: 45 minutes
SERVES: 6

(LF) (GF) (DF) (EF) (NF) (SF)

12 ounces (340g) baby carrots

11½ ounces (330g) canned whole
beets (weigh after draining)

2 red bell peppers, seeded and cut
into large pieces

12 ounces (350g) kabocha squash/
Japanese pumpkin, peeled, seeded,
and cut into large pieces

12 ounces (350g) sweet potato,
peeled and cut into large pieces

1½ pounds (700g) potatoes, peeled
and cut into large pieces

Drizzle of olive oil

A few grinds of salt and pepper, to
taste

Small handful of chopped fresh herbs
(e.g. oregano, thyme, parsley;
optional)

GINGER MAPLE GLAZE

4 tablespoons olive oil

1½ tablespoons crushed ginger*

1 tablespoon pure maple syrup

Who doesn't love sweet, sticky, melt-in-your-mouth roasted vegetables? My mom's secret weapon in the kitchen was her ginger maple glaze for roasted veggies, and she has been kind enough to share it with us.

1 Preheat oven to 375°F. Line a roasting pan with parchment paper.

2 Make the ginger maple glaze by mixing together the olive oil, ginger, and maple syrup in a small bowl or jar.

3 Scrub the carrots (halve if they are large). Drain the beets, weigh them and then cut each beet in half. Pat dry.

4 Place all the vegetables in the prepared roasting pan in a single layer and toss with olive oil. Season with salt and pepper.

5 Roast the veggies in the preheated oven for 45–50 minutes, until they are golden brown and crispy. Baste the roasted veggies with the ginger maple glaze two or three times while cooking (turn halfway through cooking).

6 Serve hot and garnish with fresh herbs, if desired.

TIPS
*Check buying tips (see page 25).

SWEET POTATO IS LOW FODMAP IN SMALL SERVINGS.

Soft Ginger Cookies

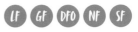

12 tablespoons (1½ sticks/190g) dairy-free spread or butter

1 cup (210g) white sugar, plus extra for sprinkling

1 large egg

3 tablespoons dark molasses

2½ cups (350g) gluten-free all-purpose flour*

2 teaspoons ground ginger

1 teaspoon baking soda (GF if needed)

¾ teaspoon ground cinnamon

½ teaspoon ground cloves

¼ teaspoon salt

1 teaspoon guar gum or xanthan gum

These cookies are perfect for the Christmas season, and a great treat to leave out for Santa.

1 Preheat oven to 350°F. Line two cookie sheets with parchment paper.

2 Soften the dairy-free spread or butter slightly, but don't melt it. Place the spread and sugar in a large bowl and beat together until light and fluffy. Beat in the egg and molasses.

3 In a separate large bowl, whisk together the flour, ginger, baking soda, cinnamon, cloves, salt, and gum. Mix the wet and dry ingredients together until well combined.

4 Place tablespoonfuls of the mixture on the prepared baking sheets (you should fit about 12 cookies per sheet; make sure they are evenly spaced). Flatten each cookie slightly and sprinkle with white sugar.

5 Bake in the preheated oven for 10–12 minutes, until the cookie bases turn slightly golden and the tops start to crack. Remove from the oven and leave to cool for 2 minutes on the cookie sheet before transferring to a wire rack.

TIPS
*Check buying tips (see page 25).

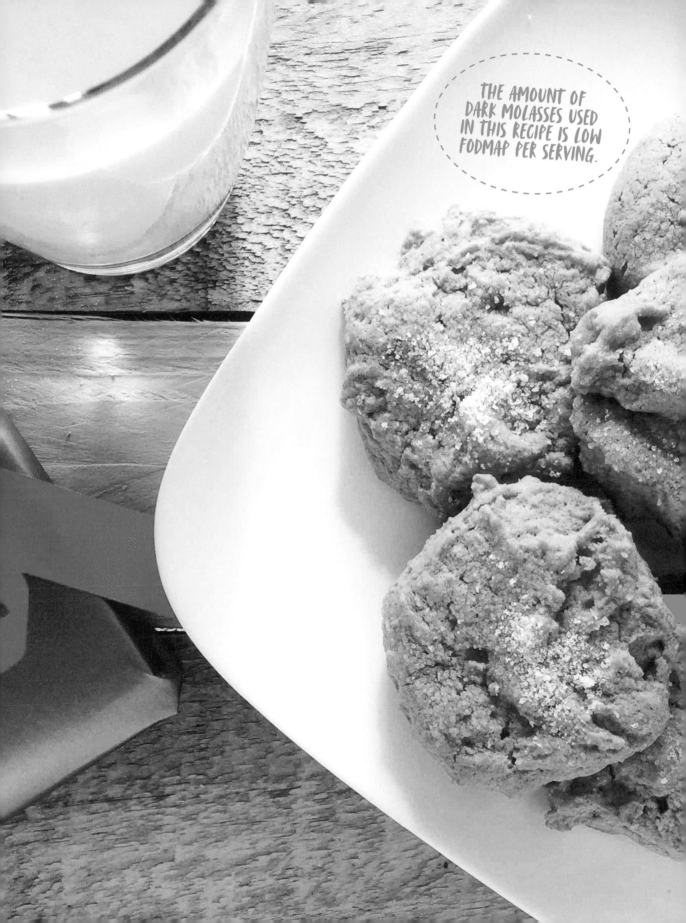

THE AMOUNT OF DARK MOLASSES USED IN THIS RECIPE IS LOW FODMAP PER SERVING.

Rustic Pumpkin Pie

PREP TIME: 1 hour + chilling time COOK TIME: 1 hour
SERVES: 10

(LF) (GF) (DFO) (NF) (SF)

PASTRY

1¾ cups (240g) gluten-free all-purpose
    flour*
½ teaspoon guar gum or xanthan gum
2 tablespoons brown sugar
⅛ teaspoon ground cinnamon
8 tablespoons (1 stick/125g) cold
    dairy-free spread or butter, cubed
1 large egg, lightly beaten
1 tablespoon low-FODMAP milk*

FILLING

1 pound (425g) pumpkin puree (or
    1¼ lb/600g raw kabocha squash/
    Japanese pumpkin)
3 large eggs
¾ cup (150g) firmly packed
    brown sugar
2 tablespoons corn starch (GF if
    needed)
½ teaspoon salt
1½ teaspoons ground cinnamon
½ teaspoon ground ginger
¼ teaspoon ground nutmeg
⅛ teaspoon ground cloves
¾ cup (185ml) low-FODMAP milk*

This is my Kiwi girl's take on a classic pumpkin pie. My family loves how it's sweet and spicy, thick and smooth all at the same time.

1 Sift the flour and gum into a large bowl. Stir in the brown sugar and cinnamon. Rub the dairy-free spread or butter (it should be as cold as possible) into the flour using your fingertips, until it resembles fine breadcrumbs. Add the egg and milk. Mix with your hands to form a rough dough. Pat the dough into a round, flat ball, roughly 1 inch thick. Wrap in plastic wrap and refrigerate for at least 30 minutes (or overnight).

2 Preheat oven to 350°F. Place the oven rack in the center of the oven. Grease a 12-inch tart pan. If using fresh pumpkin, steam in the microwave until soft, then puree and leave to cool.

3 Roll out the pastry on top of a piece of parchment paper until it is roughly ⅛ inch thick and 12 inches in diameter. If the pastry is crumbling you can roll it out between two sheets of parchment paper. Carefully transfer the dough to the prepared tart pan. Firmly press any cracks back together. Trim away any overhanging pastry and prick the base with a fork.

4 To blind-bake the pastry, cover the pastry with parchment paper. Pour dried rice or dried beans on top of the paper to hold it down evenly. Bake in the preheated oven for 10–12 minutes. Remove the parchment paper and rice or beans and bake for another 5 minutes.

TIPS

*Check buying tips (see pages 25–27).

CONTINUED ON PAGE 204

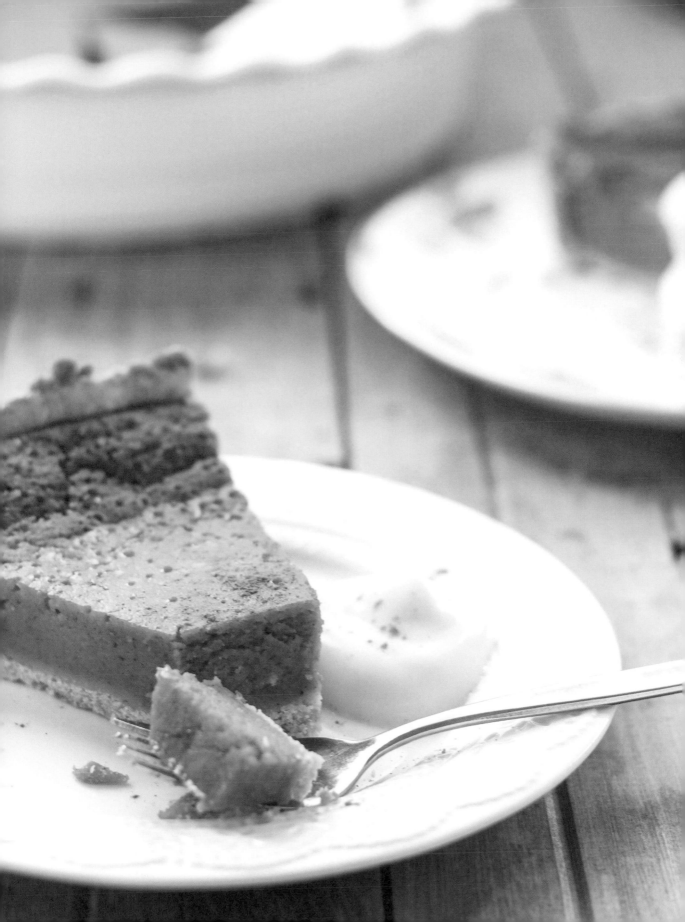

5 While the piecrust bakes, finish the filling. Place all the filling ingredients in a food processor and blend until smooth. Pour the filling into the prebaked piecrust. Fill the crust almost to the top but not right to the brim.

6 Bake in the preheated oven for 45–60 minutes or until the center is almost set (it shouldn't wobble, and a toothpick inserted into it should come out clean).

7 Once cooked, transfer the pie to a wire rack and leave it to cool completely (for at least 3 hours). Serve with whipped cream or low-FODMAP vanilla ice cream.

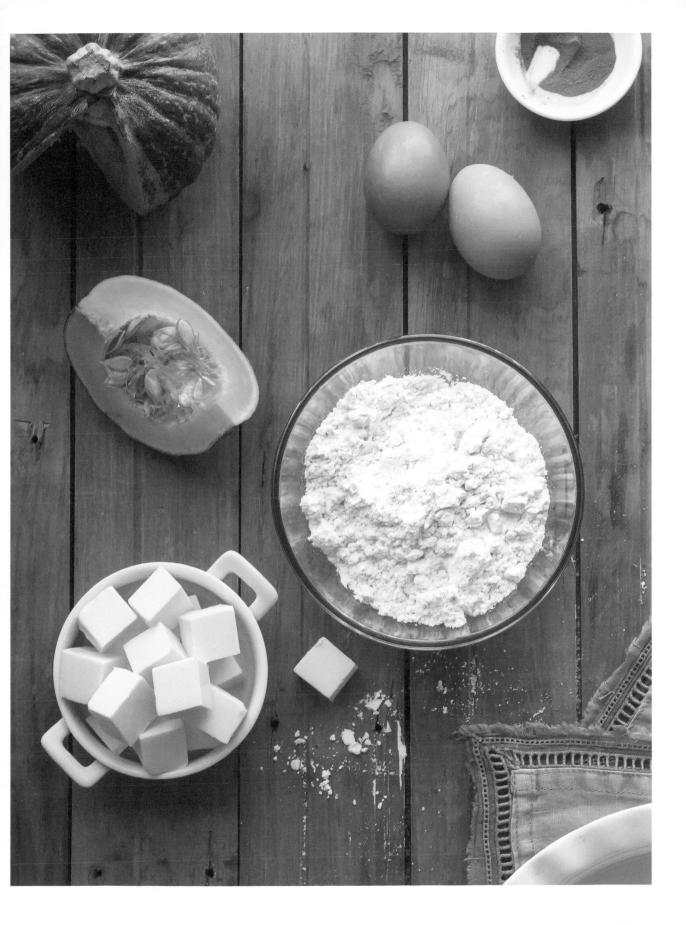

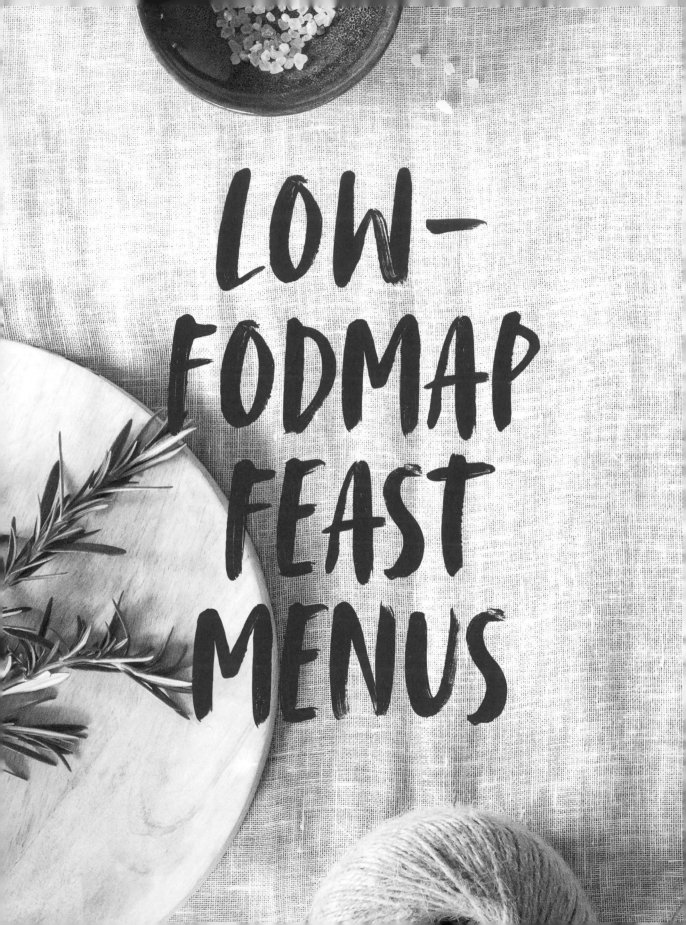

LOW-FODMAP FEAST MENUS

WINTER FEAST

Antipasto Platter	188
Roast Chicken with Homemade Gravy	104
Crunchy Herb Stuffing	194
Gorgeous Roasted Veggies	198
Caramelized Beet, Pumpkin & Feta Salad	74
Rustic Pumpkin Pie	202
Banana Butterscotch Pudding	178

VEGETARIAN POTLUCK

Sweet Red Pepper Soup	86
Crunchy Falafel	82
Crunchy Thai Brown Rice Salad	62
Magic Veggie Fritters	54
Strawberry & Banana Ice Cream with Chocolate Fudge Sauce	176
Dark Chocolate Truffle Balls	166

SUMMER BARBECUE

Basic Beef Burgers with Maple Mustard Dressing	112
Sweet & Sticky Salmon Skewers	144
Simple Potato & Egg Salad	66
Classic Green Salad with Italian Dressing	72
Lemon Meringue Pie	168

CHRISTMAS DINNER

Pork Loin Roast or Maple-Glazed Ham	190 or 192
Pesto-Stuffed Chicken Breasts Wrapped in Bacon	196
Classic Green Salad with Italian Dressing	72
Gorgeous Roasted Veggies	198
Soft Ginger Cookies	200
Berry Nice Pavlova	172

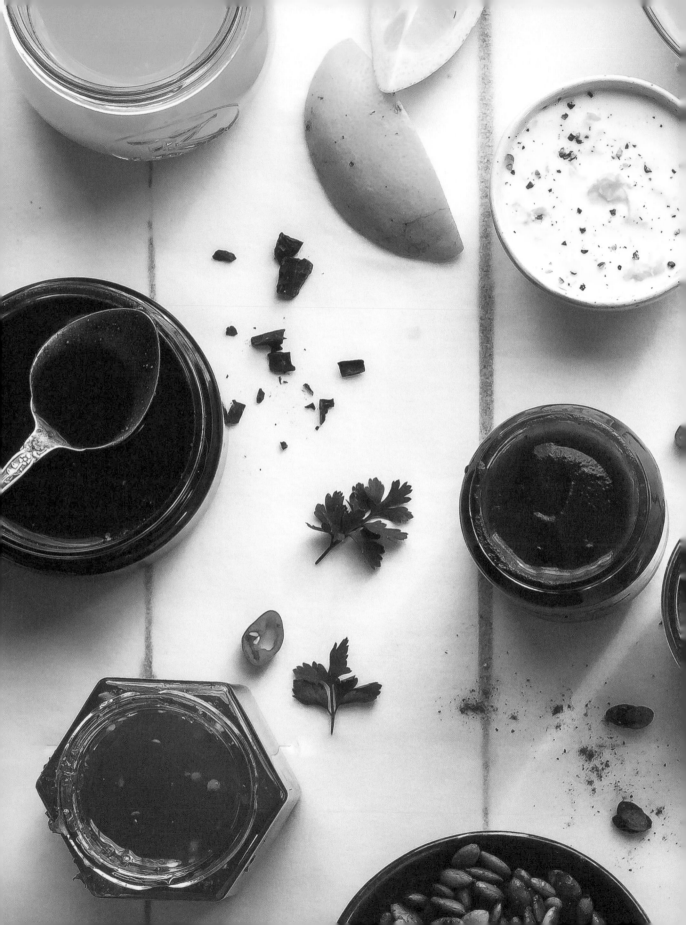

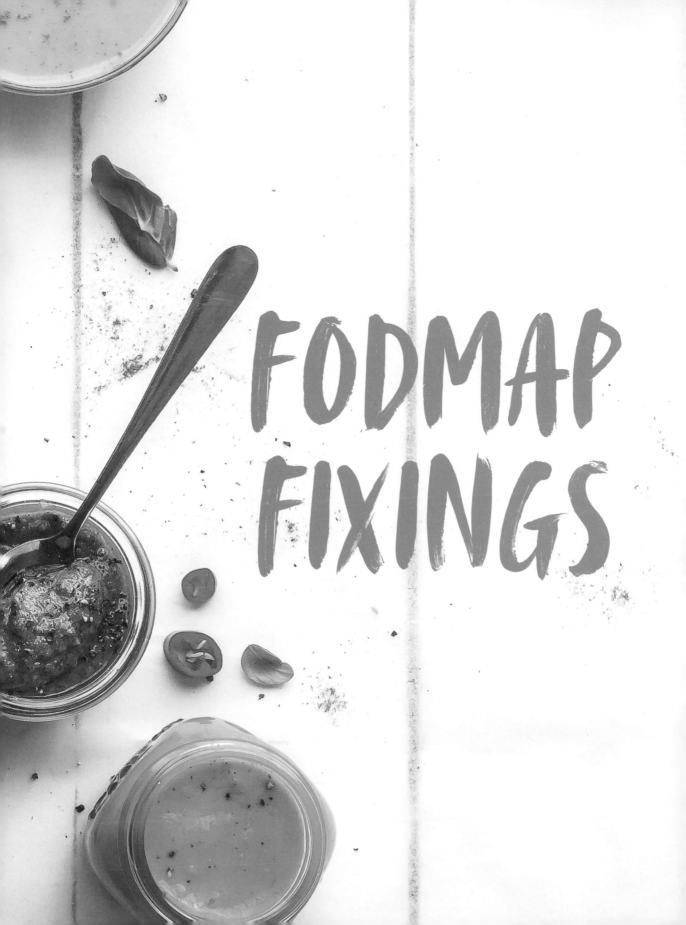

FODMAP FIXINGS

Smoky Barbecue Sauce

PREP TIME: 5 minutes **COOK TIME:** 10 minutes
MAKES: 2½ cups (limit 3 tablespoons per serving)

(LF) (GF) (DF) (EF) (NF) (SF)

1 cup (11oz/310g) tomato paste
¾ cup (150g) brown sugar
½ cup (125ml) water
¼ cup (60ml) apple cider vinegar
3 tablespoons dark molasses
1 tablespoon Worcestershire sauce* (GF if needed)
1 tablespoon garlic-infused oil*
1 tablespoon dried chives
½ tablespoon white vinegar
2½ teaspoon yellow mustard powder
2 teaspoons smoked paprika
1 teaspoon black pepper
½ teaspoon salt
Pinch of cayenne pepper, or to taste

TIPS

This sauce will keep for a month in a sterilized jar in the fridge, or you can keep it in the freezer for up to 3 months.

*Check buying tips (see pages 25–26).

1 Combine all ingredients in a saucepan. Bring to a rolling boil, then reduce the heat and simmer for 5–8 minutes or until the brown sugar has dissolved.

2 Adjust the flavors to suit your taste preferences. If you would like a thicker sauce, add corn starch dissolved in water, then simmer until the sauce thickens.

Traditional Hummus

PREP TIME: 12 minutes
MAKES: 1 cup (limit 2 tablespoons per serving)

(LF) (GF) (DF) (EF) (NF) (SF)

1 (15oz/400g) can chickpeas
    (230g drained or about 1½ cups)
2 tablespoons tahini
2 tablespoons lemon juice
2 teaspoons garlic-infused oil*
1 tablespoon olive oil
½ teaspoon ground cumin
½ teaspoon salt
3 tablespoons water

1 Drain and rinse the chickpeas, then gently pinch each chickpea to remove the skin.

2 Place the tahini and lemon juice in a food processor or blender and blend on high for 30 seconds, until well combined. Add the remaining ingredients and blend until smooth.

3 Taste and add more salt and lemon juice to suit, then blend again. Chill for 30 minutes before using.

Moroccan Spice Mix

PREP TIME: 5 minutes
MAKES: about 3 tablespoons

(LF) (GF) (DF) (EF) (NF) (SF)

3 teaspoons paprika
1½ teaspoons ground cumin
1½ teaspoons ground coriander
¾ teaspoon ground turmeric
¾ teaspoon ground cinnamon
¾ teaspoon ground ginger
¾ teaspoon white sugar
¼ teaspoon salt
¼ teaspoon black pepper

1 Mix all the spices together. Store in an airtight container. Use about 1½ teaspoons per ½ pound (250g) of meat. Goes well with chicken, fish, pork, and firm tofu.

CANNED CHICKPEAS ARE LOW FODMAP IN SMALL SERVINGS.

Slow-Cooked Chicken Stock

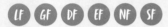

PREP TIME: 20 minutes **COOK TIME:** 10 hours
MAKES: 9 cups (up to 1 cup per serving)

LF GF DF EF NF SF

4 chicken legs

2 large (8½oz/240g) carrots, peeled and
    chopped into large pieces

2 large (10½oz/300g) parsnips, chopped into
    large pieces

1 large stalk (2oz/60g) celery, diced

1 cup (2½oz/80g) chopped leeks (green leaves
    only)

2 tablespoons garlic-infused oil*

1 teaspoon dried rosemary

3 dried bay leaves

Handful of fresh parsley

Handful of fresh thyme

12 cups water

A few grinds of salt and pepper,
    to taste

1 Place all ingredients in a slow cooker and season generously with salt and pepper. Cook on low for 10–12 hours, then shred the chicken in the stock and leave it to sit for a few minutes. Taste and add more salt if needed. It should be a beautiful amber color.

2 Strain the stock using a sieve. Leave to cool, then store in the fridge for 4 days or keep in the freezer for up to 6 months.

Zesty Lemon Aïoli

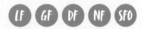

PREP TIME: 3 minutes
MAKES: ⅓ cup

LF GF DF NF SFO

5 tablespoons mayonnaise

1 tablespoon lemon zest

1 tablespoon lemon juice

½ teaspoon garlic-infused oil*

1 Mix all ingredients together in a small bowl. Taste and add more garlic-infused oil, if desired. Store in the fridge for up to 4 days.

Maple Mustard Dressing

PREP TIME: 3 minutes
MAKES: ¾ cup

(LF) (GF) (DF) (NF) (SFO)

¼ cup (60ml) mayonnaise
3½ tablespoons Dijon mustard*
3 tablespoons pure maple syrup
1 tablespoon white vinegar
Small pinch of cayenne pepper
Black pepper, to taste

1 Place the ingredients in a small bowl and stir until smooth. Taste and adjust the maple syrup or Dijon mustard if needed. Store in a clean glass jar in the fridge.

TIPS
*Check buying tips (see page 24).

Smoky Red Pepper Dressing

PREP TIME: 15 minutes
MAKES: 1 cup

(LF) (GF) (DF) (EF) (NF) (SF)

2 red bell peppers, seeded and halved
5 tablespoons olive oil
2 tablespoons rice wine vinegar
3 teaspoons pure maple syrup
1½ teaspoons smoked paprika
½ teaspoon garlic-infused oil* (optional)
A few grinds of salt and pepper, to taste
Pinch of guar gum or xanthan gum (optional)

TIPS
*Check buying tips (see page 25).

1 Grill the red bell peppers in the oven until the skins blacken, then peel off the skins and discard them.

2 Place all ingredients in a blender and blend until smooth. Thicken using a pinch of gum (or blend in a small amount of low-FODMAP bread).

3 Store in the fridge for up to 7 days.

Sweet Chile Sauce

PREP TIME: 10 minutes **COOK TIME:** 25 minutes
MAKES: 2 cups (500ml; limit 1–2 tablespoons per serving)

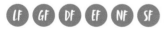

9 ounces (250g) fresh mild red chiles
1½ cups (375ml) white vinegar
1½ cups (315g) white sugar

1 Coarsely chop 2 ounces (50g) of the red chiles. Halve, seed, and roughly chop the remaining chiles (discard the seeds). Place both lots of chopped chiles in the food processor. Add ½ cup (125ml) of white vinegar and process until finely chopped.

2 Transfer the chile mixture to a saucepan and add the remaining ingredients. Heat on low until the sugar dissolves, then bring to a boil and simmer for 20–25 minutes or until the sauce thickens, stirring occasionally. The sauce should continue to thicken as it cools.

3 Pour into a sterilized, airtight jar and seal. Store in the fridge for up to 3 months.

Easy Basil Pesto

PREP TIME: 10 minutes
MAKES: ¾ cup (limit 2 tablespoons per serving)

(LF) (GF) (DF) (EF) (NF) (SF)

1 cup fresh basil leaves (tightly packed)
½ cup pumpkin seeds
6 tablespoons olive oil
2 tablespoons lemon juice
2 tablespoons garlic-infused oil*
½ teaspoon salt
¼ teaspoon black pepper
¼ teaspoon (1–2 pinches) guar gum or xanthan
   gum (optional)

1 Roughly chop the basil. Place all ingredients except the gum in the blender. Blend and then thicken with gum, if desired.

2 Store in a glass jar and pour a small amount of olive oil on top to help keep it fresh. Keep in the fridge for up to 2 weeks.

TIPS

*Check buying tips (see page 25).

Lemon Curd

PREP TIME: 5 minutes **COOK TIME:** 15 minutes
MAKES: 1½ cups

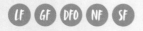

2 whole large eggs
2 large egg yolks
¾ cup (155g) white sugar
5 tablespoons (80g) dairy-free spread or butter
⅓ cup (85ml) freshly squeezed lemon juice
4 teaspoons lemon zest

1 Place the whole eggs, egg yolks, and white sugar in a small saucepan. Whisk until well combined and smooth. Place over low heat and add the remaining ingredients, stirring continuously until the dairy-free spread or butter has melted.

2 Turn the heat up to medium. Continue to cook and stir until the mixture thickens (this should take 5–7 minutes). The curd is done once you start to see tiny bubbles rising to the surface.

3 Store in an airtight container in the fridge for up to 2 weeks.

Salted Caramel Pumpkin Seeds

PREP TIME: 4 minutes **COOK TIME:** 20 minutes
MAKES: 2 cups (limit 2 tablespoons per serving)

(LF) (GF) (DFO) (EF) (NF) (SF)

2 cups pumpkin seeds
2½ tablespoons white sugar
½ teaspoon ground ginger
¼ teaspoon ground cinnamon
Pinch of ground nutmeg
2 teaspoons water

SALTED CARAMEL SAUCE

1½ tablespoons dairy-free spread or butter
1½ tablespoons brown sugar
1 tablespoon white sugar
½ tablespoon rock salt

1 Preheat oven to 300°F. Line a roasting pan with parchment paper.

2 Mix together the pumpkin seeds, sugar, ginger, cinnamon, nutmeg, and water (the water helps the spices stick to the seeds). Transfer to the prepared roasting pan and bake for 20 minutes, stirring occasionally, until golden and crunchy.

3 As the seeds finish cooking, place the salted caramel sauce ingredients in a large saucepan. Melt the ingredients over medium heat, and then cook for 1–2 minutes while stirring, until deep golden brown. Turn down the heat to low and mix in the pumpkin seeds.

4 Spread the pumpkin seeds in a thin layer in the prepared roasting pan and leave to cool. Store in an airtight container for up to 2 weeks.

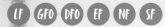

Chocolate Fudge Sauce

PREP TIME: 20 minutes + cooling time
MAKES: 1⅓ cups (limit 1½ tablespoons per serving)

(LF) (GFO) (DFO) (EF) (NF) (SF)

¾ cup (185ml) canned coconut cream
¾ cup (185ml) low-FODMAP milk*
¾ cup (150g) firmly packed brown sugar
4 tablespoons Dutch cocoa powder (GF if needed)
1 teaspoon vanilla essence
3 tablespoons coconut oil, melted

TIPS
*Check buying tips (see page 27).

1 Blend all ingredients until smooth. Place in a small saucepan over medium heat and bring to a boil. Turn down the heat to medium-low and gently boil for 25 minutes, stirring occasionally.

2 Place in the fridge and leave to cool overnight. Stir in any skin that forms on top. Store in an airtight container in the fridge for 1–2 weeks.

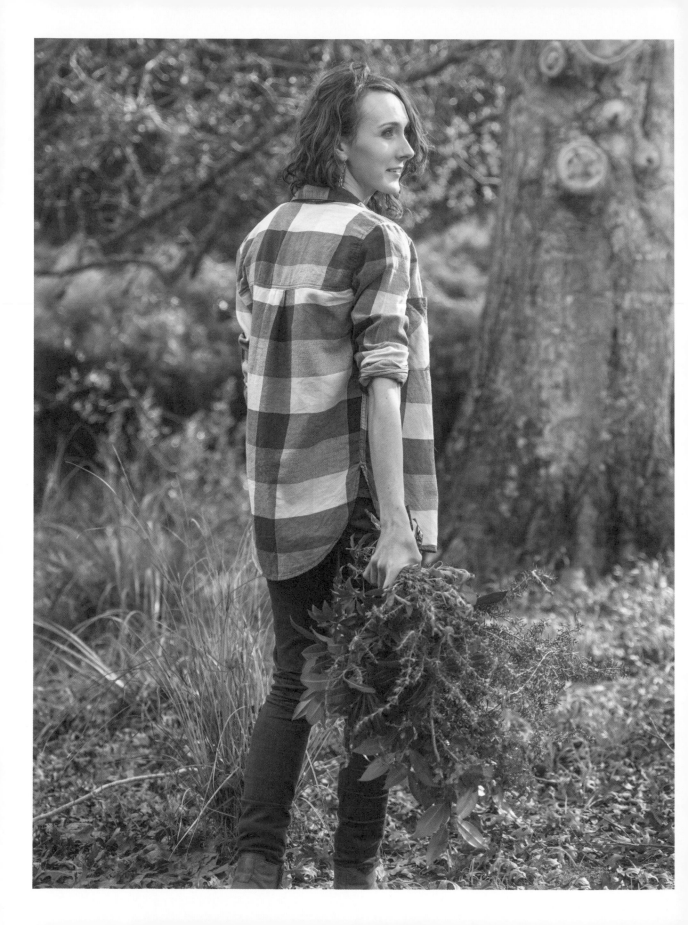

Finding Your Food Freedom

I hope this cookbook has inspired you to love your food again, and helped you to learn how to manage your upset gut. The low-FODMAP diet isn't a forever diet and it's important that you now regain your food freedom.

After two to six weeks on a low-FODMAP diet, we would expect you to see significant improvement and no longer be experiencing moderate to severe symptoms. If you haven't seen improvement, then it's time to check in with a FODMAP-trained dietitian to help you troubleshoot.

If you have seen improvement, then you can start re-challenging FODMAPs (see page 17). I know this feels scary, as no one wants to experience unpleasant symptoms. Just remember: if you do react to a FODMAP challenge food, you can stop the challenge and return to the low-FODMAP diet, and your symptoms will subside after a few days.

It's important that you re-challenge FODMAPs because they contain prebiotics that feed your healthy gut bacteria. Restricting FODMAPs, even for short periods of time, can alter your gut microbiome, which could negatively impact your health in the long run. This means that to protect your health, you need to figure out which FODMAPs you can enjoy without triggering symptoms.

Your dietitian can help you determine which FODMAP groups and how much of each food to challenge. We can also support your journey at alittlebityummy.com, through our dietitian-approved reintroduction guides, e-courses, and re-challenge meal plans. Let's find your food freedom together!

I look forward to seeing you soon at alittlebityummy.com.

—Alana
Founder of alittlebityummy.com

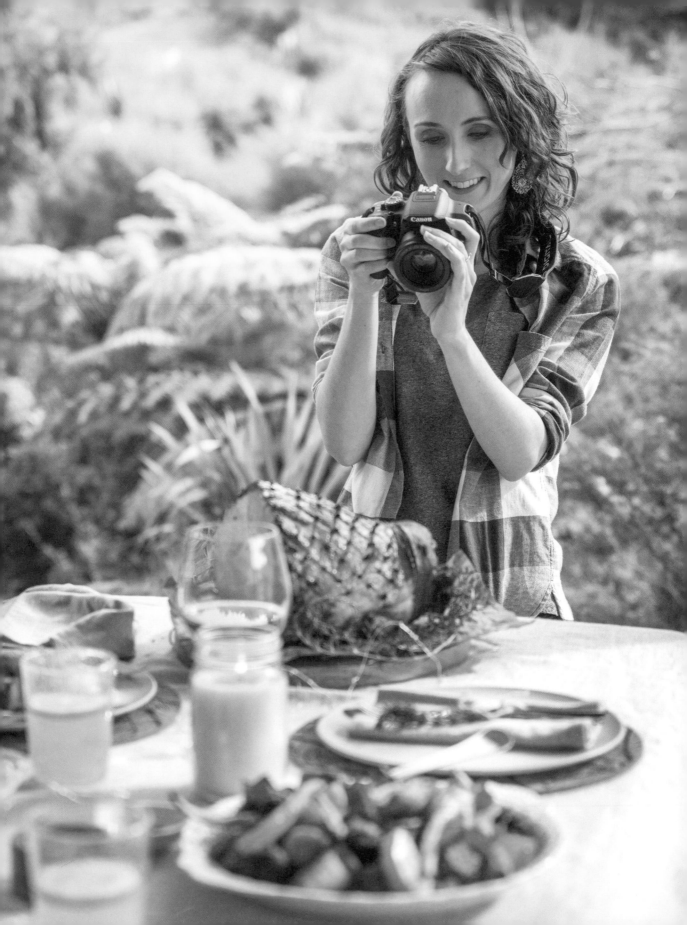

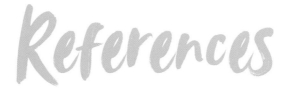

References

Biesiekierski, J.R., et al. 'Quantification of fructans, galacto-oligosaccharides and other short-chain carbohydrates in processed grains and cereals,' *J Hum Nutr Diet*, 2011, 24(2): 154–76.

BPAC NZ. 'Irritable bowel syndrome in adults: Not just a gut feeling,' *Best Practice Journal*, 2014, 58: 14–25.

Dwyer, E. 'The 3 phases of the Low FODMAP diet,' Monash FODMAP blog, 2018, 23 Jan.

Gibson, P.R., Shepherd, S.J. 'Evidence-based dietary management of functional gastrointestinal symptoms: the FODMAP approach,' *J Gastroenterol Hepatol*, 2010, 25(2): 252–58.

Halmos, E.P., et al. 'A diet low in FODMAPs reduces symptoms of irritable bowel syndrome,' *Gastroenterology*, 2014, 146(1): 67–75.

Halmos, E.P., et al. 'Diets that differ in their FODMAP content alter the colonic luminal microenvironment,' *Gut*, 2015, 64(1): 93–100.

Hill, P., Muir, J.G., Gibson, P.R. 'Controversies and Recent Developments of the Low-FODMAP Diet,' *J Gastroenterol Hepatol*, 2017, 13(1): 36–45.

Mansueto, P., Seidita, A., D'Alcamo, A., Carroccio, A. 'Role of FODMAPs in patients with irritable bowel syndrome: A review,' *Nutrition in Clinical Practice Journal*, 2015, DOI: 10.1177/0884533615569886.

Marsh, A., Eslick, E.M., Eslick, G.D. 'Does a diet low in FODMAPs reduce symptoms associated with functional gastrointestinal disorders? A comprehensive systematic review and meta-analysis,' *Eur J Nutr*, 2016; 55(3): 897–906.

Monash University App. 'Food Guide.' The Monash University Low FODMAP Diet App. 2018: Version 2.0.9(339).

Muir, J.G., et al. 'Fructan and free fructose content of common Australian vegetables and fruit,' *J Agric Food Chem*, 2007, 55(16): 6619–27.

Muir, J.G., et al. 'Measurement of short-chain carbohydrates in common Australian vegetables and fruits by high-performance liquid chromatography (HPLC),' *J Agric Food Chem*, 2009, 57(2): 554–65.

NICE. 'Irritable bowel syndrome in adults: Diagnosis & management,' National Institute for Care & Health Excellence, 2017.

Prichard, R., et al. 'Fermentable oligosaccharide, disaccharide, monosaccharide and polyol content of foods commonly consumed by ethnic minority groups in the United Kingdom,' *Int J Food Sci Nutr*, 2016, 67(4): 383–90.

Tuck, C.J., Barrett, J.S. 'Re-challenging FODMAPs: the low FODMAP diet phase two,' *J Gastroenterol Hepatol*, 2017, 32(1): 11–15.

Tuck, C.J., Ly, E., Bogatyrev, A., Costetsou, I., Gibson, P.R., Barrett, J.S., Muir, J.G. 'Fermentable short chain carbohydrate (FODMAPs) content of common plant-based foods suitable for vegetarian- and vegan-based eating patterns,' *J Hum Nutr Diet*, 2018, 31: 422–35.

Tuck, C.J., Muir, J.G., Barrett, J.S., Gibson, P.R. 'Fermentable oligosaccharides, disaccharides, monosaccharides and polyols: role in irritable bowel syndrome,' *Expert Rev. Gastroenterol. Hepatol*, 2014, 8(7): 819–34.

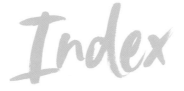

Index